Salon Therapy

Salon Therapy

✦

Lay Yo' Burdens Down by the Beauty Shop

Denise Thompson

iUniverse, Inc.
New York Bloomington Shanghai

Salon Therapy
Lay Yo' Burdens Down by the Beauty Shop

iUniverse books may be ordered through booksellers or by contacting:

iUniverse
1663 Liberty Drive
Bloomington, IN 47403
www.iuniverse.com
1-800-Authors (1-800-288-4677)

Because of the dynamic nature of the Internet, any Web addresses or links contained in this book may have changed since publication and may no longer be valid.

ISBN: 978-0-595-45731-1 (pbk)
ISBN: 978-0-595-71668-5 (cloth)
ISBN: 978-0-595-90031-2 (ebk)

Printed in the United States of America

Contents

Acknowledgments

I'd like to thank my family for all they have to help me with this venture:

Cassie, my lovely daughter who stumbled out of bed each time I messed up the computer.
Lance, who came to my aid after Cassie put me down.
Eric Junior for believing in his mother.
Eric Senior for the many conversations on being prepared and doing my homework.
Jerome, my brother, for correcting my English all the time.
My mother Lucille, for making me feel like a star all the time.
My Aunt Barbara, who has helped me in my salon for many hours.

I'd like to also thank the people who helped make sure I stayed on the right path growing up in North Slidell off Bryan Road:

Mrs. Alberta Cooper, Mr. Elijah Cooper, Mrs. Mattie Drammer, Miss Claudett Drammer, Big-Mama, Miss Kid-Lee, Brenda Power, Mrs. Grace, Mr. Mack, my auntie Fannie Mae Tillison, my stepmother Mildred Strickland, my client who has supported me through the years. Also Lucille Cousin, Francis Green, Deloris Gomez, Suzzett Faciane, Jean O'Rouk, Arlana LeBlanc, JoAnn Stiller, and many more.

Thanks to the people who helped me pull this thing together:

Miss Mary Smith: thanks a million, you're a godsend.
Leon Newsome: my business cards are great!
My poet friend, Mrs. Sylvia Brookter, a client who is truly a role model: thanks for reading my samples and believing I could do it.
Miss Pamela Daggs for *all* your constant help.

Life is a circle, and within your circle you need to keep a few good spirits. Thanks for the support.

For Frances Greene, my client-friend who always invited me into an elite world, preparing me for the day my life would change into my destiny. We always said we would take this book to Oprah!

For Katrina Mills. Thank you for beginning to write my manuscript for me in 2005. Unfortunately, Hurricane Katrina washed away everything.

Introduction

Hello, my lovely sistas and brothas who enjoy reading exciting things! Thanks for taking the time to share this salon adventure. This trip to the salon will thrill you, and it might bring tears from deep-down hurt and pain. But you'll dry your eyes to a laugh and you'll want to read more.

I want to welcome you into my daily world of hair, knowledge, and the power we possess inside the walls of what we call the beauty shop. If them walls could talk there would be some explaining to do. I want to show you the good sistas who bring good news to our healing chairs. Who have no problem with gettin' down in it for another sista. I want sistas to know that we can share in an experience not only of dislike, but also of love, kindness, and unity, that we can heal the wounds of yesterday and make your tomorrow be a good morning.

Walk through these doors, my sista. Take a seat and let the rhythm of sistahood move you to the groove of our souls uniting together as one sista.

Learn, laugh, and love. Come on in.

PART I
Lay Yo' Burdens Down by the Beauty Shop

1

Salon Therapy

There's nothing like the atmosphere in a beauty salon. The soft pastel colors bring out the soft side of a woman. Plants all around create a tropical atmosphere; pictures on the walls of faraway places let you drift off into your own fantasy. It's a place where women can come together and share so many things, whether it be how to cook a particular dish or when to catch a great sale at the mall.

Sometimes, the right picture or the right song on the radio can take your mind on its own trip, while in the background you hear the joyous voices of so many happy ladies. The salon is also a place women can get deep into a religious conversation that may bring tears to another's eyes, where you can pray and ask for family prayer. There's no limit once two or more have felt that spiritual, or just plain old sista-to-sista, connection in the salon. We may laugh and give advice on our children and school, and talk about how fast they grow up. We talk about how you're not seeing parents getting involved much in our kids' school. We talk about the difference it makes just being there for our kids.

The things we come up with in the salon to talk about: our child's first date, who is starting to get phone calls—those phone calls when we know it's someone they like, when they start that cute smiling and whispering all at the same time. We sit and express the feeling we get as parents seeing our babies find interest in the opposite sex.

Sports: that's another topic when it comes to our boys, especially the hopes of a college scholarship. It's a way to experience new and exciting things, growing and being educated all in one. Graduation is a big thing! It's so hard to believe life has gone so fast, and this child you have watched grow up is now finishing high school: it's a very proud moment when a mother speaks of her graduating child. Then there's the fear a mother feels when she must let her child grow up. Daughters spring into womanhood, sons walk into manhood, and you know they carry new responsibilities on their shoulders. This is a very painful moment for a woman; no more kissing away the boo-boo. Now it's about making correct decisions, allowing that new and inexperienced young adult to walk new paths—an indescribable passage in a woman's life.

Don't mention when we get on the husband thing' if you have one you know what I mean. Wakes up every morning, can't find his keys: like I said, *his keys,* not mine. That's what makes me want to scream—how the heck am I supposed to know where his keys are? Like I said, if you have one, you know exactly what I mean. We love 'em, but you know how the story goes.

The salon is a healing place. So many women come in with broken spirits. It's like the women at the well that Jesus met, and knew everything about them without passing judgment. There was a healing that took place. The salon is like the well in the Bible: a place where women can gather, and not only is there water involved, there's information.

Can you imagine? Back then, there was no gathering at the beauty salon, yet the well was just as important to the women there. They could share quick conversation, and they could keep up with what was going on in the city.

We know that all over the world from the beginning of time the one constant thing about women is that we love to share information, or to be real … gossip in groups.

Woman talked us right out the doggone Garden. Tell the truth now; don't get mad. Information is what we'll call it. That can save you or cost you! In many ways, it's as if Jesus passes through the salon, using sistas to give important information, information that may bring serious changes into a person's life who's been seeking an answer. It's one of the few places a woman can come and get a sense of relief. She's pampered and she has someone to listen to her and truly understand. It's different from "professional help."

Professional therapy leaves you feeling like its only you who has problems. You go into a quiet little room where the doctor sits at his or her desk across from you and asks you these dry questions. Then they sit there waiting on you to talk; they will just sit there looking at you. Over time, I guess you open up to the person. But here at the salon, everyone gets involved. They've all experienced some form of life issues and know how it changed them. Here, no one has gone to school; the lessons come from life experiences. Each person gives great detail about the subject and how they found the solution. It makes you feel connected to reality a lot more because you know this is real not just a brain-smart person sitting before you with a book-smart answer!

Many times, a subject comes up that may get so emotional, tears are wiped away. I swear, there have been times the shop has been in such an emotional state, you forgot you were even in a salon—the sistas bonding together, reaching out to someone with all the right intentions of helping a sista in whatever the situation it may be. I tell ya, if you haven't experienced a sista-ta-sista soul searching in a beauty salon, you have been missing out on who we, as sistas, really are when we bond together.

You can feel the power from within, the weight we all have carried at one time or another, the rivers we had to cross. Whether you're a swimmer or not, baby, we sistas cross 'em. Like the song, "Ain't No Mountain High Enough," that's us. We will get there.

The client speaking about the problem is emotionally involved, along with the client receiving the life lesson, explaining what she's gone through. Many times, someone sitting listening to the conversation has experienced the same situation at one time in her life. To hear it from someone else brings a vivid picture to that person along with those happy or painful feelings.

I think I saved a life one day in my salon. A client came in, someone I had never seen before and of a different nationality, yet a sister in God's eyes. For some reason, we started opening up to each other as if God himself had brought her to me. She said that she didn't know why she had come into the salon and that something had told her to. She followed the spirit. In doing so, she found out that God was going to use this little black stylist to save her life, along with the life of someone dear to her who she was caring for and had become depressed. Satan was starting to step in and cause confusion the same way he spoke to Eve in the Garden. Now he was speaking to this sista. It's funny how God works. I began to tell her about a depressing moment I'd had to overcome and how Satan had spoken to me as clear as the two of us were speaking.

One night while I was sleeping beside my husband, Satan came to me and began a little conversation. He spoke so calm and inviting; it was so peaceful. I tell you what he told me to do, and he said it so sweet, it didn't even scare me when he said it. He said, "Denise, if you take that pillow and place it on your husband's face and smoother him, when you get up in the morning and he's dead, you just tell the police that it happened while you were asleep. Tell the police you never knew you were on top of your husband." Now sista, that's the God's honest truth. Satan spoke those words to me; Satan told me what to do and how to do it. Satan told me how to get out of it. Then Satan left quietly for me to lose my mind alone!

That's when that old-time religion from my grandma kicked in. She would say, "Satan you lie! Satan get behind my granddaughter in Jesus name!" When I realized it, I was thanking God. I couldn't believe what had just happened to me.

That morning, I spoke to my husband about what had happened in the night and how, through faith, God prevailed.

For some reason, this sista came in at a time when no one else was in the salon and the spirit had me tell her this story. I hadn't spoken about this to anybody at the time, but I felt I needed to share it with her.

She looked at me and she said, "You know, I'm having a similar problem. My father has been very sick. He's old and dying and it's hard to watch. There are times I just want to end it for him."

I knew then why God wanted me to share this story with my sista. He had sent her into an unknown, unfamiliar place to an unfamiliar person to be healed from this evil, ungodly thought that Satan was trying to plant in her mind. See, Satan will plant a seed in your mind, then he'll sit back and watch that seed become fertilized and bloom into destruction while he's on the sidelines watching his garden of destructions flourish into a patch of hurt, pain, and death.

In this place you can pray and bond together with someone who has experienced your pain, and hear how the person fought the good hard fight and walked through her very own life cycle. In the salon, God's name is always being brought up; the salon is truly a healing place. There are so many women in this world dealing with hard issues daily.

The other day a client was in here, one that I enjoy doing: Mi'cka; I love her name. My girl handles business. She's been working on her job for years, handling her business, like I said! She takes her money and pays for her home that she and her two kids share. Unfortunately, she lost her dear husband to a car accident a couple of years ago and she is carrying the weight on her own. Now let me get something straight. She had a good brother side by side. They handled their responsibilities. We have some good brothas out there working hard to fulfill the American Dream; believing the vision of Doctor Martin Luther King, Jr.

I was so hurt for her to lose such a good husband at such a young age. Bruce was coming home from his son's class play when a car came and hit him head on; he was killed instantly. The complete shop just broke down with Mi'cka. We couldn't open for a couple of days. To have known that family as hard working and as supportive of their children was a blessing, especially when you see so many broken families. Little Bruce always said he was going to be like Will Smith. He was going to have his own show. So whenever Little Bruce could get the opportunity to perform, he did and his parents took turns taking off to see their star!

Their beautiful daughter, Savannah, loved dancing; she would be at the salon waiting to have her hair done. She would go outside and practice her new steps, always striving to do her best. Of course, she was highly praised by both parents.

To watch the strength this family retains, with all the deep love and devotion to doing their best, is almost unbelievable. I asked Mi'cka one day just how they went through their grieving, then pulled together. She looked at me and said, "The faith God must have meant when he said, 'If you have the faith of a mustard seed, you could move mountains!'" She said her husband had always talked to them about life after one of them had passed on. He said that the only conversation they would have in heaven had to be positive. He would say, you have to give that person something to talk about. After the family went through their grieving period, Mi'cka said she called the kids into her bedroom and they had a long talk about what they had to do so that daddy could have something to talk about! So they decided to do like Bonnie Rait said and "give 'em somethin' to talk about!" "That's what you see with my family," Mi'cka told me. "We are staying true to what Bruce said!" She rejoiced.

You know, one day after these kids had lost their father, they pulled together a car wash to help pay a bill for an elderly lady in the community. Talking about giving 'em something to talk about. That family makes you very grateful. I couldn't say one word after Mi'cka told me that story that day; I spent the rest of the day in deep thought. Something so deep, far beyond anything I could have imagined.

Anyway, back to Mi'cka. After all she has gone through, now there's a new sista on the job who has decided to give her problems. Mi'cka tells me she has tried building a relationship with the young sista. She even invited the young lady to church with her. The sista came to meet Mi'cka at her house, they rode together in Mi'cka's car, and the ride was about thirty minutes, which gave them time to get comfortable with one another. They talked about family and how they felt about religion and how important it is to keep prayer in your life. It seemed like they could be great working buddies, but when they got back to work she realized this girl didn't have a working relationship or anything else good for her.

Things began to change for Mi'cka. The peaceful atmosphere the company had once had was no longer there. Now you could feel Satan on a rampage. It was one thing or another: the supervisor was no longer friendly; she became suspicious of everything and the good relationship Mi'cka had once shared with her was no longer there. The supervisor started asking questions about Mi'cka's performance on the job, as if she was looking for an answer to something brought up by a coworker. Mi'cka kept her faith. She never once spoke an unkind word about anybody. She knew where the problem lay and she was not going to give in to Satan himself. She said a quick prayer and knew no harm would come to her. She held her head up high and stood her ground respectfully like the Bible said: "Believe in your heart the ninety first psalms. No harm shall come to you." She spoke highly of her job, had nothing negative to say about anybody, and left the office without a worry. Little Miss Mess-maker, looking all funny and, as usual, the first to ask "what's going on." "That's the kind of person you let God handle" Mi'cka said. She looked at her and said loud enough for everyone to hear "God gave me this job and what God put together no man can break. When I leave this job it's going to be because God has elevated me onto higher ground. Mark my words." Nobody opened their mouths and she went right back to work like nothing had happened. That office was very quiet the rest of the day.

The funny thing about it was that she never got ugly. She just stood her ground about who she was and how she believed there was nobody in that office who could bring harm to her, unless God was ready to move her. And she truly believed that when He did, it would be a testimony to her faith and that God would put her in a better position because she stood on his word.

It's sad when two sistas on a job can't be an example that we, too, can work and progress together. No, we've always got to entertain the company with our slavery mentality. We have been entertaining other people forever. It's as if sometimes that's all we can do together. This sista secretly resented Mi'cka. Mi'cka went to her to have a heart-to-heart talk with her. She felt like she was older than the young lady and she should be an example to the younger sista. So she decided to go to her to let her know that God has blessed her and those same blessings were open to her also. That nothing she felt Mi'cka had achieved was just for Mi'cka, and God would bless her also. That the two of them should not be on the job behaving in this manner, but instead doing whatever it took to help the other accomplish whatever goal they'd set. The young lady—who by the way is Michelle Stone—poor thing, she put her head down and you could see she didn't know how to close this problem out. Mi'cka told her she serves God because He said He would elevate His people so that others would know that the God they serve is real, and He will not forsake His own. The sad part was this sista couldn't take the sweet way Mi'cka handled things: no drama to entertain the rest of the employees. Baby, Mi'cka is so ahead of this simple stumbling block. Michelle never gave in to this conversation. Her spirit and Mi'cka's spirit just did not connect. In life it's funny how spirit knows spirit and someone can dislike you because you're a good spirit.

Let me just squeeze this in quickly: know the spirit in you. Pray that God walks with you, not Satan. Have you ever been around someone, and you didn't know what it was about that person, but you could never get comfortable around them? Their spirit just didn't mix with yours. We are spirit. The Bible says "Know the spirit and question it." Did you know you can question the spirit? I rebuke you, Satan. In the name of Jesus! My grandmother always used to say you better question that spirit—see if it's of Satan. If it is, it will flee you; if it's of God He'll answer. He'll speak to you. Know the spirit!

This conversation didn't resolve anything between Mi'cka and her coworker. The only thing that came out of this was for Michelle to start acting like she doesn't see Mi'cka, turning her head whenever their paths crossed. Poor thing. People like that make you wonder just what makes them tick. It bothers Mi'cka to a point, since she really likes people. Her family thrived on helping people find themselves through positive support in whatever way the family could help. People know that these are the families Satan wants destroyed. I've told Mi'cka how strong I see her and how happy I am to have her as a client. She just lifts me whenever she comes into the shop. This is the type of person I like having in my life: I feel it's a blessing.

Now look: Mi'cka has been blessed with this spirit from childhood. She came up in an atmosphere of daily fights. She has had her practice in it all. The difference is she knew that wasn't the life she wanted to live. Coming up like that, and hearing about the lives lost to the streets, she knew once she left that life there was no turning back. She had faith in what she believed and trusted that through faith and prayer she wouldn't bring her children up in a rough environment. She also knew this sista wasn't going to make her walk backward to prove she could be just as low down. Nope, not this sista; she has arrived and ain't going backward. So, Satan, fight by yo' self.

You know, you see people, but you just don't know what they are going through. There is a lot behind a smile. Whether faith or pain, believe me it's a story! There are women out there carrying around so much pain, yet they have to be great mothers, great wives, and also great employees on the job.

The thing is, a lot of ladies are good to everybody else, but never know how to be good to themselves, never find any time to find out what's needed for self. Sometimes I question myself in my own struggle to find peace and happiness. Do I give up so easily out of fear that I will not succeed in my own search? Will I not know how to travel into the road of my own soul and find the answers to my own dilemmas, the hungers of my yearning to find my place here on earth? To give of myself to others is to find a hiding place from my own emptiness. So when sistas come into the salon who I know are hard working, good spirited kind of women, I take my time and give extra attention to them, especially at the shampoo bowl. There's nothing like a good shampoo. It's definitely a gift when you find a stylist who knows how to shampoo a client's hair. I know from my own experience with stylists who don't have the technique at all actually. You feel worse after their sad shampoo!

Shampooing is the one thing everybody looks forward to. After a good shampoo, the client is relaxed and ready to talk. She'll fall into the calmness of the salon atmosphere and opens herself to me about the stresses of the week. You know, there is something to water. The Bible speaks about water, and the blessings that are cast upon us through water. In Isaiah, God speaks about being with you through water. In John, God speaks of the baptizing into the water. Water holds great value in the Bible and in this day and age it still holds great value. The salon atmosphere almost forces one to look at self!

The conversation that takes place, by itself, will touch something going on in your life and cause you to look at it, whether only while you're at the salon or for the rest of the day. You will look at the issue. Sometimes, someone says just what you were looking for in the salon, which causes you to want to deal with it because you know you're not alone. You realize this world is round, and we walk along some of the same circles of life. Life's track: walked by many, won by few.

Really and truly, nothing we face do we face alone. There's always someone else going through it, too. Life is a cycle, and in that cycle there are so many people rolling along on that exact track; let's call it "Life's Track." That's exactly what it is—a life track walked by so many. On this track it gets pretty dusty, but keep walking and the clouds will clear. You don't want to just stand in it! You want to keep focus and continue walking. Only in that spot will you have to come face to face with the dust. Think about it. If you stand in the dust, it gets all in your face. When you keep moving, people can't tell you've been through dust. You keep moving through it all, not allowing the dust to settle on you. Have you ever seen a person who stayed in the dust as it's kicked up? Dust in their hair, eyes, and mouth. That looks like such an uncomfortable moment, you wonder why the person didn't move out of the dust. Step back, go around to get a better view of what's going on, then walk around it to see a different aspect of this dust, but keep moving: after that the road gets clear. If you're never strong enough to put one foot in front of the other and cross over, you will never know just how clear things can be. If you grew up like I did, in the country, and remember walking down the old rock road, whenever a vehicle would pass, you hated it; dust would kick up and get into your mouth and your greasy hair. Especially if it's freshly pressed. Baby, you would have a head full of white dust. You kept walking, and before you knew it you had walked right out of the dust and into the clear—but you had to keep walking!

You remember when we were young kids, we'd go to church and the old folks would sing that old hymn, "I'm Coming up the Rough Side of the Mountain"? Well, we've made it over the mountain; God has blessed each one of us to be able to have more and also to see God-serving people succeed. To me, that's over the mountain. We have come a mighty long ways. That song, "Lord You Brought Me From a Mighty Long Ways" has true meaning. To know whatever your situation is, if you keep the faith in what you believe in, and do good works, you will make it.

If there is no one you can personally come in contact with, put that television on BET—Black Entertainment Television. You'll experience many people who were where you are, on the rough side of the mountain, some worse than you. Their end result is what matters. Through faith and good work, they are walking in God's greatness; you, too, can get there. God told us how we can walk into the life we wish to live, and the job we wish to have. He said if you have the faith of a mustard seed, with good works, he'll give you your heart's desire. Do you know how small a mustard seed is? So small you might miss it if you see one on the table. God wants you to not give up, work toward what you want, believing in Him. He'll bless you into places you've never asked for because your mind hasn't even imagined that far. Without more exposure, the brain will limit itself to the depth of your successes. Through faith and good works, all things are possible, if you believe. That's the reason I say we have crossed over. Today, our people have been blessed to bring to the table many different talents that have allowed them to do well financially in ways they couldn't even have imagined. It's like God with Pharaoh in the Bible when God said "Let my people go!" Looks like God has opened many roads for his people to travel into their dreams of success, as if he, Himself, has decided we've seen this side of the mountain. But hold on! Ya'll about to really see somethin'!

He has given new dreams to young men, new levels of knowledge to fuel burning desires. I say, dream people with forces behind the dream! I say, claim that dream with the strength of the women in Proverbs 3:25. I say, believe like Abraham in Romans 4:3. I say, work like Timothy in Romans 16:21, and your dreams shall manifest into existence. Faith with good works, manifest all things you desire! Can I get a what? Amen!

2

Headed to the Salon

Today is a sunny, bright new day! The sky is the prettiest blue you could ever imagine. The sun is casting the softest yellow across it. Looks like it would make the loveliest background for a spring picture!

The birds are flying through the air, they're sitting in trees, chirping the most beautiful morning songs you would want to hear first thing in the morning. Squirrels are running from tree to tree having the time of their life. I wonder, is this an animal holiday? I compare it to Christmas. It just looks like a happy, busy morning for the animals.

These are the days I wish I could drive forever with my windows down. I love the morning. Something is so special about a new day, full of unfulfilled dreams and desires that only you know, and each morning makes me feel like I can accomplish all my heart's desires.

The sun has blessed the world with a glow of pride, a beauty none can imitate. The trees are standing on both sides of the street as tall as green soldiers for God. The leaves are beautifully colored in shades of green, weaving from side to side, looking like they are rocking to their own heavenly beat. The wind: not too strong, not too aggressive, but giving off a breeze of gentle blessings to the body and soul. As the breeze brushes against my face, embracing me, loving me in a sweet heavenly way, bringing a calmness that prepares me for my day, I just say to myself "if it could stay this way!" I have to thank God for this free, beautiful day.

Good Morning

Good morning, I woke up early just to wish you world a Good morning!
I'm waiting with you for the sky to come ablaze with the beautiful light given as a gift from God.
He's given power over to the sun to beautify the morning.
So I wait too, to say "Good morning!"
As it lightens by the minute you can see life awaking. Its fresh and crisp, with new

challenges, new hope, and new life.
If you really sit back and allow the morning to come to you, it comes with peace,
joyful singing, and bright beautiful skies.
I bet that's why humans say "Good morning!"
A day to change your whole self and say "No More!"
For today I'm new and I'm having a good morning!

—Dedicated to everyone who says, "Tomorrow, I will!"

Headed to the beauty salon, I decided I needed a little gospel music to complete my morning. I put the radio on 94.7 FM. Bishop Paul S. Morton, Sr. and Aretha Franklin: "Season Change" is on. I turn that up, because God knows, sometimes winter looks like it stays with me a little too long. It gets rough sometimes, as if the cold chill blown from Old Man Winter just won't leave me alone. I know that after winter the spring brings new life, a bright new beginning, for new ideals and to start planting seeds of new hope, believing now that those seeds will be nurtured by God.

"Lord, I know I'm having a good morning!" The sun shines down brightly, touching me, wrapping sweet, warm love all over me, taking the chill of winter breezes away. It's a beautiful day from God and problems fade away with the rays of the sun. If you can just hold on and believe with the season's change, so is your life. I'm driving and singing. Good thang nobody's in the car with me, cause baby I am saaaanging, ya hear me?

Gospel just does something to your soul. I like to just ride and listen to my gospel, preparing myself for the day. Lord knows when the bishop sings I feel deliverance. I say a little quick prayer: "Lord, please don't let me get no crazy client today, messing up my day. It's too close to Sunday when I can sit and eat off the message Bishop delivers, and I don't want to get mad! "Season change," I say to myself. "This is an appetizer to what he delivers on Sunday morning." I start out sitting but, baby, that word has power. You gotta get up and move around. It's like those rappers Kris Kross's song that goes like this: "… make you wanna Jump Jump!" That's exactly what he does. So, let me just stay calm today, so I have no need to repent tomorrow!

Man, some of these young clients can come up in here taking up all my time with some throwed-off hairstyle she done made up with three packs of weave. Nothing like trying to understand somebody's hairstyle they had in their dreams last night! You know, one of them, "It was like this, one side was hanging with pin curls on the side and a French twist in the back with crimps underneath the

French twist." Then, she'll say somethin' crazy like, "I'm trying to get a style that go with this outfit I'm wearing tonight. Girl, it's tight!"

I'm thinking, "Lord, not today. I've just been revived; let me enjoy it today!" After you finish something this creative and challenging on a client you have spent a good bit of your time on, stressing and using all of the creative side of your brain, she looks in the mirror. The look on her face makes you want to just say, "Girl, look, if that ain't it, you've got to go challenge someone else. 'Cause baby, I surrender! That's it for me!"

She'll say something like "I like it. It's cute. I just thought you was going to make the bun a litter bigger!" Then you want to say somethin' crazy back like, "Girl, how big do you think yo' head is?" Don't get me wrong, I love creativity, but on Saturday morning, people look at me like, "I know you not!" Those looks put a stylist on the spot, you know? You be like, "Can we just use two bags of hair?" Sistas be wanting that hair. All of it!

As I pull up to the salon, other cars are starting to pull up also. Lord, these ladies are something. They try their hardest to be first. Lord knows they don't want to be behind Sista's Weave!

Horns are blowing, people screaming out the window as they pass by—always something to be said. You know how we are. I hear a yell from a car driving by, I don't even turn around to look at that crazy girl. She always comes to the shop when it's good and full, asking me to play like she has an appointment and, as always, we get into a friendly fight. Sometimes I let the cow win, she's been my crazy client for so long.

All the morning action makes it seem like a special occasion, coming to the beauty salon. Then you get one of those bring-you-back-to-reality checks: brother on a garbage truck holla out something crazy like, "Damn ya'll some fine sistas out here ta'day!" Then he say somethin' crazier like, "Now which one of ya'll I'm-a have to take out tonight with ya'll fine self?" Everybody says, "Yes indeed!" Somebody says, "If I get that bad off, somebody slap me!"

Don't get me wrong, we're not downing a hard-working brother because of his job. It's the way some men feel they can approach a woman. Real women need to be addressed respectfully, making all of us feel good first thing in the morning. More like "Good morning ladies, ya'll sure look nice this morning." We all would have shouted back something nice to him. It would have all been good. A nice "Thank you, my brother, you take care." All good, you know?

Then, he shouts somethin' crazy: "Oh, it's like that?" Yes indeed! Of course nobody wants to respond to some nut on the back of a garbage truck with no sense. He got that "yes indeed" look from the sistas, which we done perfected!

Nothing like a look of disapproval from a sista. God gave us some dangerous eyes. Yo' mama can look at you and not say one word and baby, whatever you was doing (I said was doing, cause you put a stop to it so fast, like you wasn't doing nothing), you give her that "I stop" look back quick! Them eyes get attention and respect. Them some bad eyes! Them eyes will tell you to "shut up" in a minute. No words needed, just the look. Whatever you was saying, ended immediately. You be like, "Oops!"

My clients get here thirty minutes to sometimes an hour before I open. When something is going on, like Christmas—baby there's nothing like Christmas and a woman's hair! There might not be nothing under the tree, but sista hair be laid! Yes Lord, old girl gonna take care of that head. We black women, even during your struggles, when the holidays rolled around—Christmas, Easter, and Thanksgiving—those are our days as woman, and her daughters got to have the hair done. For that day, all our problems are put aside and that day is celebrated. Even before the fancy salon, black mothers would pile up in someone's kitchen to get that hair pressed to a straightness you wouldn't believe could be. You would leave out of there smelling like Blue Magic: you remember that red can with the blue grease in it. Ears and face shining like a new penny. That stuff was good for a lot of things in the black family. Once you finished getting your hair done, you'd rub your face, then reach down and wipe your shoes and your shoes would shine. You'd look so good and you'd be so proud of your patent leather shoes.

A stylist can start styling hair as early as five in the morning for a holiday. She may not finish the last head until twelve or one o'clock the next morning. Some holidays demand that many hours, making show sistas straight. That tells you how important the beauty salon is to a sista. It is the one bonding place. But they definitely make that sacrifice getting up earlier than the salon is expected to open, with hope of being one of the first clients: get in and get out! The thing about a salon is a woman can spend her complete day in it waiting her turn if her timing ain't right. God forbid she get behind somebody getting a weave, you sho'nuff stuck!

But anyway, you get a lot of knowledge from sitting there. Either listening or sharing a few words; you never know what subject is going to come up. Sometimes it gets pretty deep.

I unlock the door, letting the clients in. Everybody greets each other with a "Good morning." Black folks, if you don't say "Good morning" to each other, something's wrong with you. Greeting is very important in our culture. So everybody coming into the salon knows to say "Good morning, how ya'll doing?" Now you can come in and get comfortable, without people looking at you like you're crazy. Trust me: go into a place where colored people at without speaking and see what the atmosphere will be like for you! Like Bruce Bruce would say, "For You!" You know, we always have one who like to be seen. She will say something crazy like, "Who that is?" "Nobody did her nothing, what's her problem?"

I remember when I was a little girl, we had a corner store we used to go to on a daily basis until we were able to go into town to make large purchases. The people who ran the store was like family—your extended family. They would correct you when you did something you had no businesses doing. On mornings, if you went into that store and you didn't say "Good morning," someone in that store, Mrs. Grace or Mr. Mack, would get you. One of them would say "I didn't sleep with you last night. You better speak when you come in here." They taught you when you was around adults, back then, they made sure you had respect for each other. As I said, back then, adults talked sense into you. No high education, but enough life-taught knowledge to carry you. I don't know why this ritual has gone on so long, or why if it's not done it offends people. People in our culture will let that mess up their day. Trust me, next time those same people see you again, they will remember you didn't speak and they will not speak to you. They'll say something crazy about you to another person like, "I don't like her. She act funny sometimes, so I ain't got nothing to say to ha!" Trust me, it's said. But I can tell you we are growing as a people anyway. You just better remember to speak! Yo' mama could be done had a heart attack, and you grieving, you better stop grieving for a minute and nod yo' head a little bit. We understand nodding as hello also. That's so funny. I guess we are some unique creatures.

Once you're pass the greeting part, now you can relax until you're called, check out each other to see who's got that magic hair bag: weave! Weave in a ladies hand is like the monster in the shop; nobody wants to be behind that person. Lord knows we all like a little weave, sometimes. Weaves are a very consuming thing that can turn a woman from a short hairstyle to a beautiful full-headed style. It can be a beautiful thing. Now, like with everything, some people overdo it and the end result's horrible! Again, like Bruce Bruce would say, "That looks good on you!"

My salon offers bonding weave, which is applied using bonding glue and normally lasts a client about a month, depending on the client's lifestyle. Another method I use is to braid the hair to the scalp, then sew the weave to the braids. Once hair has been applied, I cut it to the client's liking and style it, making a sista feel real good. You are ready to go somewhere once you look into the mirror. You know when you done hooked a sista up, she pull out that lipstick before she get out your chair! Sista feel good! Yes indeed! She can sashay now! What that rapper say? "It's going down!" I love to watch my sistas transform from the sista who walked into the salon into the sista who walks out of the salon; it's something to witness. Sistas take on a new personality. She know she straight, her hair's hooked up, she put her a li'l lipstick on, got her earrings back on. Now, it's all good. It's like, "Lets do this!"

3

Hey Ya'll, Come on in

I turn the light on and let my clients flow in. Out of respect to the people who showed up early, I make it a habit to ask them to sign according to how they pulled up to the shop; that way nobody gets upset about the sign-in book. I get them set up, then I turn the music on, oldies but goodies playing. Marvin Gay is singing "What's going on." Somebody says, "My weave!" then she holds up a bag of hair and we all laugh and say together, "You gonna be straight in a minute!" See the night before a sista is to come to the beauty salon the sista gets her sleep on. She done slept on her face for days, she done laid on her hands trying to keep that hair looking good! That's something sistas have in common—we try to keep that hairstyle as long as we can. Sistas pay good money for these styles. Baby, they try hard to keep these styles in: they want all their money's worth.

It's funny. We took our kids to Disney World and there was a sista there I happened to notice. Her hair was cute, pinned up really cute. You know, when we go on vacation we don't want to be fooling with no hair so we braid it or pull it up; well hers was pulled up. Her head must have been itching, she was just'a pattin' and beatin' her head. I said to myself, Lord, no matter what part of the world we travel sistas gonna protect that 'do. She was not scratching and pulling at her head no matter how much it itched; she was not trying to mess her hair up.

It make you wonder when was it ever said how to preserve a hairstyle. Or is it something in our black genes, this gene that automatically triggers the hands to go up with a rhythm so good it relieves the discomfort. Only hairstylists notice these things, I know. Hair in the black community is truly our glory and it represents you even when you don't know you're being checked out. Normally, if your hair is just downright looking good, somebody's going to let you know. They will come up to you and tell you how nice your hair is, and they always want to know who did it. That's the best advertisement, because that person see your work, and they will try you at least once. That's why a stylist has to be on top of the different styles coming out.

Now you know the flip side to that story. If the head is tore up, then you know the deal. Sistas, when your hair looks like you never heard of the invention of the comb and brush, don't leave out the relaxer, you're doing real bad; it just looks like you don't care. Hair is like your first introduction as you go anywhere: job, mall, anywhere outside yo' home. If that hair isn't neat, as a woman you just don't look kept at all.

Now let me be a little funny. Have you noticed these sistas can pull some good-looking men sometimes? Have you ever walked through the mall and seen this fine-looking brother with this tacky-head looking woman and wondered, "What the hell is going on?" Man looking so good, passing by smelling good, nice clothes, just everything in order. What the hell he sees in that tack-headed female? You walking and another female make eye contact with you because you think the same thing; you both smile and shake your head like, "What the hell!" Sistas always wonder if brothas scared to approach a woman with herself together. Brother be holding hands with the sista, just all over her. So those of us who are aware, and chose to not belong to the bad hair club will sit, and wait until we walk out of the salon hooked up!

This sista walked into the salon. Beautiful lady. She wore her hair full and up high on her head, looked like a very classy lady. Makeup on every spot on her face, jewelry on both hands, sista is sharp! I'm like, "Hi, how you doing, can I help you today?" She says her stylist moved and she was in need of a good stylist, she had seen my work on a lady at church and thought she'd give me a try. She said, "I heard good things about you." I thanked her and offered her a seat. She of course said hello to everybody and took a seat. She looked so good I had to tell her how nice she looked. One of the customers agreed, saying she wished she could look like that early in the morning. Of course, everybody agreed saying, "I know that's right." Mrs. Thang had it going on and she introduce herself to me: Mrs. Barbara Johnson. She seemed like such a pleasant person, soft-spoken and not demanding in any way. She smiled and began small talk with the other women. I looked up at the clock and the morning just went by so fast, which always means I've been doing some heads.

The sun is truly hot and sunny now—good and hot, another one of those hot Louisiana afternoons. My client tells me to put extra hairspray into her hair since it's so hot. That's Louisiana for you; living in Louisiana you learn to get that hairspray! Sitting around, we start talking about the mall, of course. that place makes a woman lose her mind. Betty brings up that Mervyn's has a shoe sale. Now, most of us need to stay our butts out of the mall. Yes indeed, Mervyn's always have a good shoe sale. I hate to walk into the store because when you park outside of Mervyn's and go in you have to pass the shoes. Before you know it you have a pair in your hands to put on your feet—oops! We do some advertising for that store, so you know now where I'm going after work: straight to the mall—I'm-a just look! I'm not going to go in the mall and lose my mind up in there when I realize how much I've spent. Why couldn't I be Oprah, just for one day, to just cut loose? I have a good heart; I would think about others, yes I would. You know shopping releases something in a women's body that gives a burst of happy energy that brings so much relief for that moment: "Spend money, cry later!"

Anyway, back to Mrs. Johnson. Sista looking good: big hair like your more mature elegant, seasoned women. She has her makeup on so beautifully. She has jewelry on both hands. Sista is sharp. I'm like, "Mrs. Johnson, you're comfortable, I'll be with you shortly." I have to tell her she is a pretty lady and her age is definitely not doing her any harm. She smiles. There's nothing like being able to give a compliment to another sista, especially when you see a mature women who's kept herself so well through all that life sends out.

I've styled my last client's hair that's ahead of Mrs. Johnson and I'm looking forward to doing her hair. I've learned in this business, and any other hands-on business, you tend to attract people who represent who you are. Pleasant people tend to attract the same type of people. I've always strived to be the best I could be with my clients. I like the fact that this client carries herself well. Many people allow life and the many challenges it introduces to wear on them. Not this lady: life brought it on, and she handled it. These are the clients that teach young women how to keep their head up even during the storm of life!

She sits in my chair and we talk about what she wishes to do with her hair. She's talking and I'm enjoying my pleasant client. Here we are in the salon alone, so I'm able to give her all my attention and let her see from her one-on-one experience with me that this is where she wants to continue coming.

Life has funny timing. Suddenly, oh no, here comes my most crazy client, and I never know what's going to come out of her mouth! You know, everywhere you go there's the sista who just don't care how you see her. As they would say, "Ain't nobody doing nothing for me up in here so I ain't worrying about what they got to say, I'm taking care of my business!" And trust me, they mean just that: taking care of today is all that matters to them. They see life in a different picture, to them it's a dog-eat-dog world! Class is the last thing on their mind, more like gettin' theirs, as they say. Poor Sonya come in all loud: "Girl, what's up?" Then she say, "Oh hey, how ya'll doing?" She catches herself before she cuts loose.

Mrs. Johnson says hello as pleasant as she was when she came in. Sonya ask about her hair, wants to know, can I take her today before I close. I say, "Sure, that won't be no problem."

I joke with her and say, "Hot date?"

Why did I play with her like that? Sonya with her crazy self turns and says, "He ain't my man but I'll let him spend a little money on me." She laugh all crazy and say, "Girl, I gotta handle my business!" I say to myself "That's what you get; you asked and you know she gonna tell it like it is!" As she walk out the door I tell her to come back in about three hours. She turns and says, "You getting; ready to put a workover on her," then walks off. That child is funny.

I've known Sonya for a very long time. I think that's why she comes to me: she's comfortable here, and knows I'm gonna let her be herself regardless. There've been times when I've had someone in here and shes asked "Who that is, she seem stuck up," or she'd say "All your clients stuck up." I think she's just uncomfortable with their strength, and the fact that they hung in there and did something with themselves. It reminds her she still has to do something different in this world to live a better life. So I think for her, seeing them makes her see herself, which brings her pain.

As she walks away, poor thing, she's got on shorts that are too short, leaving nothing to the imagination, and a top that just covers her breasts and ties in the front. Its not like she has to dress like this to get attention; Sonya is very attractive. She has the most beautiful mahogany skin you've ever seen. Her sable eyes are very mysterious, and she can pierce into her target's soul. Her cheekbones stands out high and beautiful. Her one problem is that she has not valued Sonya in a healthy way. Her life and the things she's been exposed to have not allowed her to see that she is worthy of anything she sees one of these other ladies with. Without a guide, or any direction into the proper way a lady does things, a lot of Sonya exit. Unfortunately, she doesn't know the value of loving herself, and respecting herself.

Sonya gets into her car and pulls off, and Mrs. Johnson says, "That's a nice-looking young lady," not saying anything negative about her at all—not that I expected her to.

We picked up where we left off before Sonya came in. Mrs. Johnson is wearing a sewed-in weave. She does not like the way her hair feels when she touches it, and she doesn't think it was done correctly by the last stylist. I take her hair down and look at it and I understand what she means. The tracks are too wide, and you can feel lumps on her head: she definitely doesn't want to feel those tracks. That's the difference between a good weave and a not-so-good weave: the way it feels and falls into the style correctly.

I know the feeling. One day, I tried a new technique on myself, applying the tracks on the crown of my head a little differently. I doubled the tracks and alternated forward, then backward with the direction of the weave track. The look was very pretty but I didn't like the way the bulkiness felt. Well, as usual, when you do something new, something else new comes up. I had to go to the doctor, who wanted me to have some x-rays done. Trust me, I was looking good: my hair was looking straight; one thing I can do is hook up my head. Girl, when that guy touched the top of my head I could have died right there!

Trust me when I said died, I mean *died!* It played over and over in my head: did he feel my tracks? Why did I do my hair like this? Oh Lord, I can't believe it: this man touched my head.

Believe me, you trip like that for a while. So yes, it's very important that the weave is correct! You have one of those Keith Sweat moments: "run yo' fingers through my hair, and love me down." Well, after them fingers go through that head the love me down would have been gone!

He would have been like Marvin Gaye: "What's going on?" I have to laugh at my crazy self sometimes when I see some of this jacked-up work, and the crazy stuff that comes to my mind. Of course, I can't share these thoughts with my clients, so I be on my own little trip—tell Mrs. Johnson, sure, I can take care of her. We both laugh: it looks like she understands all my crazy thoughts! Sorry to say, I knew exactly who'd done this work without Mrs. Johnson saying one word. I've seen a few of these victims before! Hair weave victims on the salon run! Now, look, Sista, "stylist" is a name that can make you or break you. Learn to say these few words: I'm sorry, I'm not as talented in that area, but I do know someone who could take care of you. Don't be afraid of losing the client. Trust me, she'll respect you more with the truth and the fact that you was honest with her—she'll be back to you. You'd be surprise how much respect you'll get in the long run. Every professional person has to have a network of people, or else you end up with this!

They didn't just come up with the saying, "Just say no!" This was not a saying just about drugs, Lord no, it applies to so many more things, and this is one of them! I've got to make sure I take care of Mrs. Elegant; she definitely doesn't deserve this hair drama. No romantic moment will happen with lumpy hair: you'll wonder, can them tracks be felt? That'll mess up a night right there. You're worrying the whole night: Lord, please don't let him touch my head! The other one we stress over is can anyone see the tracks? Tracks can sometimes be so wide-looking, like railroad tracks, inviting Amway to come right on through!

Mrs. Johnson asks, is it possible for me to redo her weave with thinner tracks? She liked her hair very full sitting on top of her head, looking like one of those women on T.V. You remember Diana Carol? Mrs. Carol was always together; she had it going on in her days. Anyway, I tell her "Yes indeed, I'll take care of you."

I love doing weave; there's nothing like it. You go from no hair, or say less hair, to this beautiful head of hair, looking like those super-growth hair grease commercials, with hair down your back! We used to spend some money on some super-growth hair grease; we wanted some long hair. Now we ain't thinking about no super growth grease, we want to know, "Where the weave at?" It creates the image we as little girls just could not get: hair the length and color we wanted. You could have been just as ugly growing up, but if you had naturally long, healthy hair, people liked you, and you had all the little boys. Just as ugly as sin, but you had that hair!

That hair was something back then—people had no problem calling you "tack-head" quick. If you didn't comb your hair, you got called "tacky-head"; someone would be saying something to someone and they would say something like, "You know that tacky-headed girl, or woman." In our community, we're known by the head!

We can now have hair as long as we want; whatever color we want, its there.

Now let me say something very important to a few sistas out there that truly need to read, "I Know Why The Caged Bird Sings" by Maya Angelou. Some of us still have some childhood hang-ups about being a blond: we've got to let go in some cases!

See, we as women can see a sista with a color that is totally wrong for her, that actually takes away from her appearance, but we all know we can't just say, "Baby, that hair ain't gettin' it!" Now you know what they call that in our culture: hatin'. We just don't take constructive criticism without finding a reason, other than the truth, why you gave it. You just got to be hatin'.

It's funny: I remember a sermon by my copastor one Sunday, before Hurricane Katrina destroyed my home church in New Orleans East, Louisiana. Copastor was speaking about sistas and brothas speaking to one another. She spoke on how important it is to just smile at someone. You don't have any idea what a smile can do for a person who may have had to fight Satan to get to church.

She always gives good, sometimes funny, examples. This one was truly funny: she said, "Now look, sistas, just because you got a new weave don't mean you too cute to speak." She say, "Walking around with your head so stiff like you gone mess up your hair if you say 'hello.'" She gives true examples that we must respect. Sistas, it's not that serious. God has blessed us with new ways to improve ourselves, but let's not let carnal things like a weave cause us to miss Heaven!

That stuck with me because I know people like that. I be like: I hope she haven't forgotten we go way back and she ain't never had no hair. Just couldn't grow no hair, even when Jeri curls was growing everybody's hair, she still couldn't grow no hair—now she tripping. Those are the type of people you want to pull out their high school picture and say, "excuse me!" Trust me, that's all you'll have to say to get her straight. Sistas, lets not go there. Take your blessing and be grateful!

Weave for a woman is as bad as Viagra for a man. It makes you lose your mind. Gonna bust hell wide open, gonna be down there asking the Lord, "Lord, why you let me get this weave in my head? I went and lost my mind! I should'a known I wasn't gonna know how to act." It's a shame how a weaves make a sista trip. They literally change personalities, from the sistas I knew to Mrs. Thang! Lord don't let them get no contact lenses: I don't think their mama can't tell them nothing! Now that makes me say, "don't be hatin' on poor Michael Jackson, 'cause some of us change everything we can afford." Some of these newfound women would change their skin: wouldn't be no dark folks 'round here! Don't let Michael Jackson's doctor start no layaway plan. I can see it now: storage room full of nose, lips, and breasts, be looking like an *X-Files* movie in there. You know most layaways have to be paid off before Christmas. Be a long line of sistas getting body parts, so leave Michael alone.

I know how important a weave is, 'cause let me tell ya', I'm a Hurricane Katrina survivor, and let me tell ya', I didn't know how important a weave was until everything was closed and I had nowhere in Slidell to buy me some weave. My hair was a mess; I had been pulling out all the furniture and stuff that was destroyed. Yes, I looked a hot mess. My nappy hair underneath my weave was rough; I couldn't make it another day. I got into my car and my destination was anywhere that sold weave. God was on my side. I drove by a Beauty World and saw that door wide open letting the place air out. I pulled up to that door like a weave robber. I said to the Vietnamese man, "Please tell me you saved some hair!" He said, "No electric." I said "Don't worry, if you have some, I'll pay cash just give me some hair." He come back with some black weave, and I grabbed that pack like it was oxygen. I don't think I waited on no change—I had my carnal blessing in my hand. I thanked the Lord and drove home like I had precious cargo with me. I threw the weave in the back seat and it landed in my grandkids' car seat. I said "Oh well, if the police stop me, I can make them laugh and say something crazy like, 'at least my hair is in a car seat.'" Sometimes a good laugh keep you from getting a ticket; the way I was driving I needed some quick answers just in case.

Now you know it would have been a mess if somebody followed me home for my bag of hair. You know how crazy we get: girl see something like you got the last pack of weave, whatever it may be, 'cause humans are straight-up crazy sometimes. I get out of the car, sista behind me jumps out the car running up to me for my bag of weave. Lord it would've been somethin' in that street. You know how they say give 'em what they want. I could not have done it. My boys are ultimate cage fighters and I think everything I've seen them do I would have done to that poor hair robber.

Hair was important to me at that moment in life. I just couldn't take it one more day; life had kicked the hairstylist butt. People may say, how could you be worrying about yo' head at a time like that? Honey, let me tell you, I looked so bad weeks after Hurricane Katrina. My life consisted of digging in mud, walking in mud, eating with flies something I thought I could never do. Smelling death in the air, of wildlife and whatever else that didn't make it. One day I passed a mirror and what I saw scared me. I needed just one clean day because I had became not a soul sista but a cave sista. I was losing it that day. I said to myself, today you got to pull it together, just for today, 'cause I was in that war zone of survival with my mass destruction look on, fa' real.

A news crew was on my street and I looked so bad I ran from them. My mama said, "Girl, they would have gotten you some help, once you would have been shown all over America." I said, "Yes, that's possible, but the way I was looking like a mad hairstylist gone wild I would have been the talk of town right here." It wasn't pretty. I said, "See, Red Cross should have had a hair drive." Can you see it along with the food they was serving? You could have gotten you some donated hair from those sistas that didn't use the whole pack! Like I said, "Save some." See, times like these we can afford to help a sista out. Trust me, your day may come and it's those little things you rely on, that have become important in our lives.

I thought to myself as I was pulling boxes of stuff out of my house, I though, Lord, they gonna know all the black women houses, weave just strung everywhere by the street. I had to laugh myself, than I bent down and put my wet hair deep down into the trash. See, that didn't make it on *Dateline*, or *Oprah*: how many sistas was out there looking rough and in need of some hair. I know Oprah had some unwanted bags somewhere, between her and Gayle they could have done a little somethin'. And don't leave out Star Jones. We'da been in okay shape down here in Louisiana. I'm not going to leave my white sistas out: Pamela Anderson and Britney Spears could have hooked ya'll up. You know I'm saying all this, you know the one good thing about weave is it has helped our little girls that just could not grow hair at all. I don't care how much you greased the scalp, prayed over it that hair on some of those baby's heads, it just would not grow! So here comes the weave invention, the one way a little girl can have a pretty ponytail.

See, back in the day when I was growin' up, we didn't have weave, so when we played around the house imitating folks who could move or shake the hair on their head, we had to use a towel or anything that could hang from our head. Child, it used to be something else, our imagination was something. I don't know why one of use didn't invent the weave—we was on it. One day when we were kids, friends of ours was at my mother's house. The kids was much younger than my brother and I. Well, the young boy loved this little nappy piece of hair that used to hang from the back of his head. Correction: it didn't hang, it was just balled up back there. Back in the days people called it a tail. They would try to make a ponytail out of it; now some people had it going on with their tails. Some people should have never thought the idea up. Well this was a case where that tail used to drive us crazy. One night my brother cut the tail off the little boy's head.

Lord, why did he do that? That child went crazy; he screamed and threw a fit! When I tell you he went off, you can't begin to imagine. He went psycho on us. I was like, oh we done did it now. Man it was one of those "Lord help us for we know not what we have done." This eight-year-old is about to commit murder on own our teenage behind. I was young but I was on to something. I told my brother to glue it back—that was the only way we was able to stop that kid from cuttin' up. He was dead serious about his tail. To this day we laugh about that until tears roll down our face. We, or should I say, *I* was on to something, I don't know how long it stayed in his head but he stopped crying and having a fit while he was with us.

Now look my, non-Afro-American sistas, this is an inside secret we share in our sista-hood. See, you read our books and get some juicy, funny never-forgetting info. I ain't joking, girl, I laugh myself, and I just love us. We were girls gone wild before the saying was popular! We have been blessed to be able to add a beautiful head of hair to our pretty little girls' heads.

Now sistas, let's not get crazy with the weave. Some of these kids have so much hair on their little heads. I don't know how they hold their head up. Remember, too much of anything is a sin! I think they need to add that rule to

Sunday school teaching. "Thou shall not put all that weave into thy daughters head least yea shall be brought before the church!" Maybe that thought will stop someone who feels they have to use all the hair in the pack. "You don't: its not food, it won't go to waste!"

Girl, I feel a weave drive coming on. Somebody in this world can use that left-over weave. You remember years ago, this black sista was kidnapped in Iraq somewhere. They had her give a speech and her braids needed to be redone; that sista was so worried about her hair. I remember how she looked terrified every time I saw her. I felt horrible for her; I thought she was scared to death. When that sista got home one of her first statements was "I was worried about my hair." She wore braids and I could see it was time to have them redone. Child, I don't know, I think I would have forgot I had weave in my head, but she didn't. Being on national news, sista was still worried about that head. You know what community she from: the one that will call you tacky-head. You know it!

I was so happy to hear that, because it meant the sista was still in control of her mind, they didn't break her down completely. Sistas, I'm telling you, a few packs of weave could make the difference even in a war zone: fight all night, braid hair in between shooting, in daylight do a couple of braids. Donate the hair! Send those gift boxes full of all types of hair.

Have you ever seen a sister who didn't have enough weave to cover her complete head so you see all her little tracks showing or you see her rough hair sticking out without enough weave to blend and hide the bad stuff? Well, this is a case where she needs a donation! Now look, sisters, you know we crazy. We don't walk up to no sista talking 'bout no, "Here, I thought you could use this," and give her your leftover pack of hair. Oh no, 'cause first of all, you hatin', cause yo' hair don't look like that. Second, who you think you is? Third, no you didn't! Here's what we got to do: have a weave drive at the salon, then the stylist will recommend something cute. That way she's not so offended. 'Cause you know we still kind of sensitive about the hair thang.

Imagine what these poor white teachers must go through, especially if they're not a science teacher, used to worms. At the end of the day, hair everywhere, little braids everywhere, looking like earthworms. Poor science teacher thinking all her little earthworms done got out! "No, its just a little girl's braid done fell out." Now me with my crazy, scary self, my mind be elsewhere. I walk up to a braid that fell from somebody's head, I jump. My mind be thinking it's a baby snake or sum-um, only to realize it's someone's hair! Its funny, you walking in a parking lot, somebody done lost his or her little braid. Women kick it or pick it up, don't let folks see our mess! Some things only we should know!

Back to Mrs. Johnson. Thank God she ain't reading my crazy thoughts. People say I have this ladylike look about me. I smile and thank them: God they don't know how crazy I can be. I start working on my client, cutting these tracks out, taking my time not to cut any of her natural hair. Her hair is so pretty; it's a soft texture, pretty silver hair blended in all the right spots looking like highlights. Her hair is so long you can tell it was once nice and thick before life and all its issues took their toll. Leaving memories of what was. Thanks to a nice weave done correctly, she's still hold on to yesterday's look—just these days she holds a classy, elegant well-seasoned look. This lady still has it going on!

We talk about me and my family. She asks all those questions about my parents. It's funny, her husband teaches at the college my son attends. She mentions how many years her husband's been a professor at the University of New Orleans. We talk about the excellent education the college is known for. I can tell she's pleased to hear something positive about a young black family.

She speaks highly of the life she has been blessed to live. She attended a small Catholic college up north were she met her husband and his sister. She became good friends with Tammy Johnson. Little did she know: she and Tammy would become family.

Graduation night, she met one of Tammy's twin brothers, Michael. Michael was a very handsome young man. A quiet, mysterious young man, he had a very sexy way about himself—not pushy but direct. He asked Barbara if she would have lunch the following day before his family left to go back to Louisiana. All the rest of graduation night she says she was a nervous wreck, trying not to show her family how excited she was. For one, her brother would have teased her the whole night. She and her brother was very close. He was two years older than she, but he always stayed close to her even when he went off to college.

Mrs. Johnson looked so bright telling me about meeting her soon-to-be husband. When she told me about her date with Matthew it was as if nothing else mattered. I could feel her joy and it was a wonderful feeling, her thinking back so many years as if it was yesterday. The look on her face was worth millions; she wouldn't give up those moments for nothing. She told me he was her first real date. She had never really been out alone on a date with a guy; she always brought a friend along with her. That day was just different. She felt it and so did he; this was the beginning of forever between two young people. The closeness they felt as he touched her hand—very gentle and very respectful, making sure to treat her like the lady she was. They found themselves laughing as if they knew each other forever. Michael asked her about her dreams, where she wished to be in the future. After she told him about her plans, he came out of the blue and asked her, could she squeeze him in there somewhere? She played like she didn't hear him, only for him to repeat himself, looking directly at her. He was very serious; he knew exactly what he wanted and he wasted no time—she was for him! She thought her stomach was going to explode, she said. When she was able to speak again, she shyly answered him with something crazy like "Where do you live?" After she said it she felt like, "Why did I say that?" Michael was very patient with her. He knew she was so nervous because he just smiled at her and said, "I will live wherever you live, I have to see you again." She never answered. He knew her answer from the way the air was and the unspoken words that came from her eyes.

Mrs. Johnson made me laugh when she said, "Girl, I wanted to run out of there screaming. That man made me crazy." I thought that must have been something because she seemed to almost become youthful just talking about it.

I love to hear my more mature clients talk about their past. It is so clean and respectful, different from the way life is today. This is one of the good things about being a hairstylist: you get some good touchy stories that you can just listen to forever. All said and done, Mr. and Mrs. Johnson was planning a wedding two months after meeting. The wedding was a Christmas wedding and it sounded so beautiful. Her bridesmaids carried beautiful red poinsettia bouquets and wore the most beautiful emerald green dresses you could imagine. The guys wore black tuxes with black ties and handkerchiefs the same color green as the ladies' dresses.

The church was a winter wonderland for any child. It was the North Pole itself, just white scarves hanging from everywhere with the tallest Christmas trees in each corner of the church. I thought to myself, this lady has it going on because back in those days you didn't hear of no wedding so creative. Mrs. Johnson was everything she looked and I was pleased she choose Reflection of Beauty, Hair Salon. She shared with me the type of job she had, a job I never ever considered. It's a job you know someone has to do, but I just never met anyone with such an important responsibility. She studied babies born with abnormalities. Sadly, she said I would be surprised at the way some babies are born. There was a case she worked on were a baby was born with two heads, one fully formed, the other not completely developed. The baby didn't live and after the funeral services the parents donated the baby to the hospital for study. Sometimes these babies go on to live a healthy life. Once the child goes through intensive surgery, then a good plastic surgeon comes in and removes the scars and disfigurements and make this baby as normal as possible.

This was truly an eye-opener, and a "be grateful" moment for me, acknowledging how much I complain and feel I don't have the things in life I deserve.

This moment says, you have life, and a blessed healthy one. I have to give thanks to the Almighty, for I know through his mercy and grace he allowed me to have my health at this time and didn't use me as an example. In the Bible God said he formed the blind as well as sight, so I say, thank you, Lord for my health. I know all things have a purpose and good is in it all. Nothing is done for pain. I know God used Job, his most trusting and faithful servant, to show Satan that through it all Job would keep his faith, and that's exactly what happen. Through it all Job believed. When God blessed Job he multiplied what Job lost and the world watched as faith prevailed.

I just thanked God he blessed me with healthy children, not because I was so special, but because he used someone else's life as a testimony. Mrs. Johnson said when she got ready to have children it was very difficult, but through God she had her family—three girls, no boys: Mattie, Mary, and Monica. Each one's married with families. Each one gave her grandsons to add some men to the family along with healthy granddaughters. I tell Mrs. Johnson her job makes me feel so meaningless. She said, "Oh no, baby, it takes a lot to do what you do." She said "What you do with your hands, making nothing into something wonderful, is amazing." She said, "Then you listen to all these people's conversations, good or bad; that's something psychiatrists charge for." If you got paid the price a psychiatrist charged you'd be rich, 'cause you hear and help out a lot of people that walk into those doors." I laughed and said, "Well, I'm a salon therapist!"

I had just received my new title, which is truly well deserved. Mrs. Johnson says "You should be called that instead of just a stylist because you do so much more to a person. Their inner self is medicated when they leave out of here."

She says, "I know you hear some things!" I tell her, "Yes and in my chair it's said, and in my ears it stays. I'm like Vegas: 'what goes on in Vegas stays in Vegas!" I think after being around my grandmother, who shares the same name as one of Mrs. Johnson's daughters, Mattie, I learned a lot. Back than when we was kids, adults talked to you all the time—as they said, "talked some sense into you." Well, I was the type of kid who needed a lot of sense talking for some reason. I think what was said not to do, I did it. My grandma would say, "This little Red-Girl always try me!" I knew what that meant: go get a switch, you gonna get a whooping and a talk. They would whoop yo' behind and preach to you about what God loves. You always wished they didn't have a long sermon while they was whooping yo' behind.

Then it would be the days when she would talk to you about life, which was always a warm, loving good talk. Those talks stay with you in life and when the time comes and you need to go within yourself and find an answer they are still there tucked away, waiting on you. Now as an adult I know how to communicate with anybody, regardless of age. I know how to make sense of things. Most of my clients tell me all the time they love to talk to me. I'm the type of person who gets involved in the problem to try to make a difference. I never want my client to leave with a problem if we didn't try to work on it through talking, or if there's anything I can do I will to help someone.

Anyway, back to Mrs. Johnson. She had a lot on her mind and needed a neutral person who knew neither party that this conversation was involving. She didn't live in my community; she wasn't part of my simple little world. If she hadn't come into the salon I wouldn't have known her or her husband. I was lookin' at her in the mirror and I could see the expression on her face that said, "… that I've come to know so well." She needed to talk and she needed to let out a lot and now! Her whole proud and all-about-me expression just left. She started looking like this humble little girl with so much confusion, pain, and all those things that break you down to feel lost and alone. The look on her face I knew so well; I've seen it walk through that salon door over and over again.

Life is a puzzle. Every day you get a new piece that just don't seem like it belongs. That's how life is; it comes without a picture or directions, and it just comes. Like a puzzle, nothing is familiar, but then it fits and you wonder just how it didn't look like the other piece. Once it's in the right place, honey, it will fit. We normally wonder why we couldn't see it clearly, or the other thing, why we didn't follow our first mind. Normally God warns us, being the humans we are, we tend to question our first mind. The old saying follow your first mind, it's of God; then we go do totally opposite. That's how life is, the same way; nothing is with instructions. No warning signs, no one to blame when things go wrong.

In life, issues come with so much pain we choose to not accept what's happening. We allow the pain to slap us in the face over and over again. Instead of a black eye you receive bad nerves, hair loss, and a lack of sleep. A lot of times you find yourself putting on stress weight or losing weight from nowhere. These symptoms turn into very serious illnesses that can leave your life in a disabling situation. Stress is the number one silent killer; each year people die from some form of stress related illness. That old saying, "You look like you been in a fight!" is a true statement being made without acknowledging the true meaning.

We are in a daily fight to survive the struggles of life. We fight to smile every day, we struggle to say, "Good morning" to one another daily. Feeling so torn many days, we struggle to go to that job that no longer gives us a feeling of accomplishment.

4

Caught up in Illusions

It's funny how conversations always begin as if it's all about me. "So how you doing?" the client always asks me, knowing all along it's about to be open session for them. I always try not to complain, knowing there's other things this client really wants to talk about, knowing my problem is far from her mind. I ask the same opening question about her, how it's been for her. This normally opens the door for the client to feel free to let it flow.

Before I could get myself ready for the conversation she just came out with it! She's carrying so much pain she feels no need to start out slow. She say to me, "You know, my husband had been doing things I never thought he would ever do. He is no longer the man I once knew." She says she doesn't know what to do with the situation. She puts her head down and says to me, "Those people called "strawberries," well some kind of way he has found himself spending unhealthy times with them." Her tone is so soft, the tone of a sad little girl needing her mother's warm arms around her, holding her grown baby and squeezing away the sorrows.

I'm thrown; I almost had to catch myself. I say, "Excuse me," 'cause this elegant, classy all-that-I-want-to-be woman cannot be telling me what I think I'm hearing! So many questions popped into my head, like, what the heck are you telling me? Don't destroy my perfect picture of you and the life I believe you live. You seem to have everything I've been dreaming. Her appearance gave off such a lovely story of togetherness, stability, and happiness!

She says "I'm sorry, I shouldn't be telling you this stuff, baby." I'm like, "Oh no, I'm all right. I hear so much in here; you are just one of the many people I try to help feel better while they're in this salon: as I said, I'm a professional salon therapist!"

I ask her, "What makes you think your husband is doing these things you're speaking of? You just don't look like you would have those problems. You are just everything a man needs: classy, sophisticated, educated and beautiful, pleasant personality, all this in one person. I could see if it was just beauty you offered him; no, you offered everything a man should be proud of in a woman."

I asked her is she one of the women of excellence? She said, "It's funny you asked that. My girlfriend belongs to a congregation where the women are call "women of excellence. She's always trying to get me to come join in on some of their functions." She says that since I mention that, she must check out what's going on over there. And me not knowing her friend's been telling her about the group of women she felt Mrs. Johnson would work well with. It was like a confirmation, which God always gives you when its true. Mrs. Johnson thanked me for the description I gave her of herself. My pleasant and caring ways toward her was perfect for the way she was feeling, at the moment and in the past few weeks of her new discovery. I just had to ask her, "Why would he chance losing all this? For what? Why, what the heck is going on in this world when a lady of your caliber is dealing with this problem? Ya'll should be truly enjoying life and all that it offers. All the good fruit of ya'll's labor, beautiful grandchildren, traveling and walking, reminiscing on all of yesterday's memories."

I felt so hurt, so let down—not only for her, for myself also. Where is the American Dream, the going to work, doing what it takes to be able one day to play together off the fruit of your labor?

She just looks so much like the dream, Mrs. Cinderella in the flesh if you allow yourself to dream. She goes on to talk about the late-night adventures he goes on, or the fact that he just don't show up after work—something he never did; he was a very consistent man. As a woman, we all have that intuition we feel when something isn't right. It's time to pay attention to your other half and his actions. As women, we will be sitting down watching a movie and something will say, "Go look in the room under the rug behind the chest; I swear you will find something every time."

So Mrs. Johnson got one of those intuitions and looked into the trash can and of course she found what she was hoping she wouldn't find. It was a receipt that he must have forgotten to throw away while he was out. The address looked familiar but it was a part of town they didn't travel to, so why did he have a hotel room in that area? There it was, right in her face, so she had to find out the truth! One night he left the house and she decided to follow him. After all, he was her husband and she felt like this thing had to come to an end.

One night Matthew came home from work and he seemed kind of distant and irritable, which is not the kind of person she was used to: her husband was kind and loving, asking how her day went. So today was the day to take the challenge on, head on as they say. As I said, we know when something is up! Mrs.

Johnson's mind was made up and nothing was getting in her way. So as it went he had to make a run for a moment and without waiting on a response, he was out the door. This time, guess what? She was out the door behind him. She said she hopped into her car, which is a beautiful gold Lexus. She said she turned the radio off because she felt so nervous, hearing the radio didn't help. When you're nervous and under stress like this, seems like everything just bothers you. She's driving behind Matthew's Cadillac truck as he turns left, and she turns with him. Mrs. Johnson was hoping this thing was not real. Maybe, she thought to herself, he just needed a place to clear his head. A place where he could go, not too expensive since he just needed a place to get away for a while. Afterward he would return back to his beautiful gated community along the Lake Pontchartrain Shores.

There had to be a reason for this situation. This was just out of his character the way her husband was behaving. All kinds of crazy stuff went through her head. Lord, maybe my husband's been sick and he comes here to get some relief. Maybe he's helping someone who doesn't have a place to stay and he's footing the bill without worrying me with it. I know how kind my husband is to his relatives and friends. This has got to be the reason. Then she said she starts praying, "Oh Heavenly Father, please Jesus, let this be something I can deal with. Lord you know my heart is good, I help everybody, I pay my tithes in the Church, I follow your word. Lord Jesus." Mrs. Johnson said she never felt so lost before. She kept on praying: Lord, please don't let Satan test my marriage, my life, and my faith, which is my everything.

As she was finishing up her prayer, Matthew's truck stopped in this not-so-kept neighborhood. Not to be judging or criticizing the community, by no means. God has blessed me with parents who believed knowledge would bring us out of those situations. Not that you're better in any way, it's more that you paid the price it took to stay out of this environment. They're hopping into her husband's car. She was this sad-looking thing of a woman. Hair hadn't been combed today, and here it is late after hours: hair looking as if she didn't own a comb! Poor thang, she kept looking around nervously as if she was waiting on other people to come running! She scratched her head than scratched her arm. Poor thang, Mrs. Johnson thought, and "maybe he's helping her." After all, the man I married is a good man and he would help her if she asked. She's fighting to hold on to that. Then the girl got into the car, and as he pulled off it seemed like nothing else mattered in this world. The air seem to stop blowing; there was a buzzing in her ear, she said, that got louder and louder. Her breathing got deeper and deeper. She said it felt like she needed an oxygen tank. Her eyes became focused on nothing but that car! The Lord had to be with her because she couldn't have been driving that car herself. It was like those signs on the front of people's car that read, "God is the driver." She said "It had to have been His grace and mercy that kept me" because as she passed those eighteen-wheelers on the highway she did not see them nor did she feel herself steering away from anything. It was if she was in the car looking out at her husband and lost all sense of care or concern about her surroundings. At one time, she said, she remembered gripping the steering wheel so tight for dear life, she realized she was squeezing so hard her hand began to hurt. She just could not loosen up on that wheel. She was breathing like it was her last breath! Sweat flowed down her face. She looked over to see if the air was on, feeling like she was about to pass out. Passing out was going to have to wait; she said she didn't have time for that. Today was her day to bring this mess to a close. A truck passed by, blowing its horn to bring her back out of whatever she's in. She throws her hand up like, "I'm sorry," but the man still looks at her like, "Fool, get out the way!" She knows the driver is saying, "She done lost her mind." "Little does he know; yes I have," she says to herself. "I'm focused on my husband's car and right now that's all that matters. My complete life is fading away from me." One minute her life is as perfect as it could possibly be. A bright husband's everything you could possibly desire. He had treated her as sweet and loving, as you would a precious jewel.

He's educated, had put himself through college, and now he's a professor at one of the top universities. He has the respect of the community. He has everything going for him.

He even helped men coming out of jail find their way back into society by helping them get a general education diploma and find employment. He's a good man. He donates all his used suits to this cause, and is always available to help in many other organizations in the community. "This night is not making any sense. It just doesn't fit into our life," she thought to herself. Or was she talking out loud? She didn't know what was happening at this strange moment. I think to myself, my grandma used to always say little sayings to get us to understand. She wasn't highly educated from any school, but knowledge she had. Those old sayings in her words were so true and they could always help you when you found yourself in situations like these. She'd say "Look, Baby, everything you see ain't what you looking at!" Or she'd say, "Everything look good ain't good!" and "So don't be looking at other folks and what they have, you live life the way the good Lord meant for you!" Right now I understand what she was saying. She'd say "'Cause you gon' get their problems right along with it!" I truly felt sorry for Mrs. Johnson but I was grateful I didn't have all her glory and her sadness. This poor woman: I can't believe she could or would be going through an experience like this. I say to my long-gone grandmother, "I hear you loud and clear!" You just don't know what people might be going through.

5

When Dignity Ain't in It

Her husband pulls up into this little worn-down motel. She's thinking, "Okay, he gave this poor thang a ride, so now she'll get out and he'll be headed back to the house." No, he pulls into a spot and parks as if he'd been there many times before. "I watched him" she said. He seemed very familiar with his surrounding. The girl jumped out of the car and it looked like every move she made was very sharp, no smoothness whatsoever. She got out of the car as if she wasn't used to riding in no car, slam the door. It's something about a person that don't have a car; they always slam your car door as if they're not used to closing no car door—it never fails. She said every time she gives one of the younger family members a ride somewhere who has never had a car, they always get out and slam that door. It's like, do you have to slam the doggone door every time? You feel like screaming. So as Mrs. Johnson looks at this girl and she slams the door, it almost makes her laugh. If it wasn't such an serious situation she would have, of her prediction. "As I drove behind the two of them I could see the poor thang just'a moving around in the car. You could tell she had problems. How could he ride on side of that and not come to his senses and say, 'What am I doing?' and get out of there? She'd look out the window, then she'd jerk around and say something to him, scratching the whole time a kind of nervous movement where you just do it to be doing something. Poor soul was like something you think they made up on television. She's playing this role as if she's Halle Berry in that movie, *Losing Isaiah,* only this was real, Lord, as real as it gets."

"This was happening. My husband and this crackhead: "strawberries," as they call them. They're there together, a situation that, if I hadn't decided to see for myself, I wouldn't have ever believed."

I sit there and hear all this word for word. Believe me, I hear some stories but this detailed story I just couldn't believe; it was making me just totally shocked, just thrown. I pulled myself together as she sat there quiet for a moment, nobody saying nothing. I guess she couldn't believe what she was saying to me and why. I had to pull together all this info. That quiet moment helped me 'cause I needed a breathing moment. I think my mind went into its own defense: it truly didn't want to accept what she was saying. I stood there not knowing what to do or say, my mind playing tricks on me or trying to save the pain of reality. It's saying to me, in defense of the illusion I got from my first impression of Mrs. Johnson, "Maybe the man is trying to help somebody. After all, he is a good guy. I think to myself, he does help the men in the church with their good causes. He just can't be out here doing wrong, not from where he's from. I think, see, the devil done got this woman to follow her husband and all the man was doing was helping somebody.

Mrs. Johnson interrupts my little train of thought and goes back to finish her story. She says, "The two got out the car. Matthew walked fast toward a door, as if not wanting to be seen with the young lady. She dragged along toward the same door and as she walked she was just 'a-stretching and looking around like, I spy something. As they went into the room, which he had a key to, Mrs. Johnson said she got out of her car and just stood there for a minute not knowing what to do next. She knew she would never cause a scene or bring any attention to the situation. This was truly something no one else needed to see nor know! Opening that car door was like opening your loved one's closed casket. The pain was so great, words could not describe the feeling. She pushed it open with all her might. Now Lord, she thought, now that the door is open, will I have strength to stand? She threw one leg out the door and it seemed like hours had passed before the other leg followed. She took a deep breath to just allow her body to float up, as you do when you swimming. She just didn't feel as if she could pull this hard dead body up. As she stood there she felt like she had just arrived on the moon. Her steps were none she had ever experienced. She felt as if she was floating, yet each step was so heavy. She walked to the front of her car, than turned around and walked toward the back. Now what am I doing here, she wondered. She almost forgot her reason the pain was so strong but within seconds her horror was once again revealed.

She began to walk toward the room. This was one of the longest walks she had ever taken in her life. She didn't know which walk was the longest, walking up to her mother's casket at her funeral or walking toward this door that seemed like it kept backing away from her. It was almost as if something was trying to save her from any farther hurt and pain. But the truth was; nothing but God could ease whatever it was she was going to walk up on.

She began to pray: "Lord, strengthen my mind for the truth, strengthen my body for the blow, strengthen my heart to carry the burden that it's about to bear." One foot continued to go in front of the other until she found herself standing at the door where her husband and some person unknown to her were. She though, should I knock? No, maybe that wouldn't be right, especially if he's only in there to help this poor girl. Should she call his cell phone and see just what he'll have to say about his whereabouts? As she was about to think of something else to do the answer came to her. She could see that the curtain was open enough to see inside the room and the lights were on. This short walk, too, seemed like it to took forever. Her heart was beating so fast and loud, she thought to herself, "I won't have to knock. The noise my heart is making is going to cause everybody to open their doors." She got to the window, closed her eyes, and said to the Lord, "Lord you said you wouldn't gives us nothing we can't bear! Now Lord, I stand believing in your word that whatever happens you will see me through."

Slowly, she opened her eyes, and to her amazement there stood the man she married, pants down to his knees, and the little sad thing down on her knees performing oral sex on him. There he stood, eyes closed as if not wanting to see the sin he's taking part in. She didn't want to see anymore and forced her legs to move away from the window and bring her to my car. How she made it, she did not know, but as she walked she remembered the poem, "Footprints in the Sand" and felt some strength.

"I made it to the car and sat down inside still not believing this night and the activities of it there in that room a woman is bring pleasure to my husband using her mouth as if he was a lollipop or something, he looked as if he could barely stand up. She took his whole private part and put it into her mouth like a stick of gum. He holds her head with both hands looking like he's having a heart attract."

This filth, shame, and hurt feeling of failure she knew she did not deserve. Nothing she could have ever done to anyone would bring this hurt on. She sat there waiting on the Lord, for there was nowhere else she wanted to, or could, turn with this information. After years of turning to her heavenly father—as the old folks would say, "Lay yo' burdens down by the riverside"—she knew when she brought the problem to God she wouldn't have to hear it being repeated again. She prayed and prayed until she forgot where she was. When she came to she started up her car and left with an empty heart and soul. The one thing she knew was that God had her problem and she was going to wait on him to deal with it. She said, "I knew that he was going to lead me in the right direction to heal me from this pain. God puts people into your life to bring you answers to questions you've been praying about."

Get Behind My Brother Satan

Ole Satan you've been busy. You've walked the world and taken so many of my
brothers' souls.
Get Behind My Brother Satan
Satan you've made my brothers do things they wouldn't have never done.
Get Behind My Brother Satan
My brothers have lost all the strength and dignity of a warrior.
Get Behind My Brother Satan
Tears from their mothers' eyes have mopped the floors.
Pain from their hearts has made so many doctors rich.
Get Behind My Brother Satan
Their wives who once knew a man, and grew to love, no longer have him.
Their kids cry to just sit in their presence.
But our brothers are no longer there.
Get Behind My Brother Satan

—Dedicated to: Lost men—we still have hope for you!

God works in mysterious ways. You'll wonder why you're talking about a particular subject, but the truth is God is working something out through that conversation. Mrs. Johnson says she drove on home, but this time she knew God was with her because she had just felt his presence and knew he would carry her through! Now let me explain to you all who don't know what a strawberry is. She is the sad sista that's been through so much hell in her life that she gives in and allows herself to be used by the streets and everybody else who sneaks into the dark streets to live out some sneaky fantasy. Used by so many men until she no longer values herself. She turns to drugs and alcohol to drown out her own scream for help. Remember, this is still some mother's baby. Her mother's home worrying what's going on with her child. It makes me think about the song "If You See My Child." The song says "If you see my child somewhere as you journey here and there, tell her I'm waiting for my child to come home!" The words to that song bring chills to me: I think of all the mothers worrying about their child. So many mothers have lost their sweet child they once knew to the disease of the streets. The pain that they know their child carries, and all they can do is pray and wait on God to move that. He will, but in his own time. God uses people for his own purpose, and plain as he used Job in the Bible, he still uses people for his purpose.

My Grandmother used to say "God moves when he's ready." She'd say, "His time is not our time." When God moves its well done—that we know and trust. See, when God used Mary Magdalene to wash his son Jesus's feet, he knew just who he was using. He knew she had been through some things in her life that others never forget. But when God is ready to wash away your sins He'll do it in the presence of those who like to judge others, as if they themselves are perfect. God used Moses. Do you know that Moses killed a man? God went to Moses and used him to speak to Pharaoh. So we must remember to judge not by what our eyes see but to remember God is in control. We must thank him and be prayerful for others, not pass judgment as if we're white as snow.

Mama Didn't Know I Cried So

Woke up this morning feeling that same deep feeling. Washed my face only to
look into the mirror and find a tear, see
Mama Didn't Know I Cried So
I tried to stay busy throughout the day.
Mama Didn't Know I Cried So
That deep feeling controlled my head. I tried to laugh out loud, and act proud,
see
Mama Didn't Know I Cried So
That night came so slow, a time to be alone, less laughter, less talking.
Time to be real and that deep feeling swept into my head, it cause me to cry.
Mama Didn't Know I Cried So

—Dedicated to: Women on the streets. God hears your cry. He is waiting to hear
your voice saying, "Here I am Lord!"

The song I was talking about says, "Lord, my child may be somewhere on his sickbed with no one there to rub his aching head. Lord, my child may be somewhere in some lonely jail with no one there to pay his bail. She say's if I only knew what town my child was in I would be there on that early morning train, no matter what's the price. Lord you know that child is mine and I'm waiting for my child to come home." It's a sad song and sad situation to be in. Leaving families hurting and praying for God to deliver there love ones. It's a lot of sad mothers along, sad wives that have to deal with these sinful men who use these ill women to do the dirty sexual things, only to receive a few dollars for a drug habit.

This client sitting in my chair dealing with this problem is not just some simple little somebody. This sista's got it going on, or should I say, looks well put together. She tells me she knows the community thinks she's well off, happily married, living the life people her age who have prepared for this time in life are living. This lady had the look; she had what every women her age would kill for. Her makeup was beautiful—not too heavy, just the right amount to bring out her best features. She had the prettiest dark eyes, the way she out lined them with smoke eyeliner, with just the softest shade of burgundy. She'd applied just enough mascara to make each eyelashes appear to be speaking a unique language of their own. Her lipstick was the prettiest crimson color, making her skin glow. Her skin was so pretty she didn't need any foundation, just a little power to soften her already beautiful skin.

When I tell you God blessed this lady with the beauty, she was truly blessed. She wore the most beautiful rings on her fingers. Not too many, just one on each ring finger. Those rings were so beautiful that was the only two she needed: no need to apply one to each finger; these rings carried their own. Her bracelets dangled around her wrist, beautiful yellow gold embroidered with white gold. There was a lovely tennis bracelet that looked like it was a couple of karats. She dressed in a beautiful Liz Claiborne casual pantsuit. Her shoes you could tell she paid good money for. Mrs. Johnson looked like what we all think a woman with a good life and money should look like. For some reason we are all blinded by material things. We form our opinions from what we think we see. All along this sista is suffering more than the lady on the streets. I guess you say, how is that? This sista doesn't use drugs to bury her pain every day; she wakes up and faces it. Drug free, alcohol free, she feels all the emotional cuts, slaps, and humiliation, and so many other things words just can't explain! I just let her talk. You can tell she's hurting and dearly needs a friend—not even a friend, just some ears. I'm always that person: a set of ears and a comb. There is no pill like it!

6

In This Chair, Let There Be Knowledge

I start off by having the client sit in my chair, place a cape around her, then grab my comb. I stand behind the client asking questions. Before you know it, honey, I done put the comb down. I'm now standing there with my hand on my client's shoulder, shaking my head in disbelief. Tears try to form up in my eyes for her; I push them back. I tell myself, "This client needs me to be strong. She needs a strong listener—now don't you fall to pieces with her." I decided to give her a poem I wrote that I knew would help in her time of storm.

Looking Out My Kitchen Window

Looking out my kitchen window, God began to talk to me. There stood an old oak tree, Beautifully standing there the way God meant for it to stand.
The moss hung from the branches giving it the Old Father Time look.
I stared at that tree, because God has always given me love for trees; see, trees represent life.
I began to hear God say, "Look at that beautiful tree, It stands so strong. Full of character from many years of weathering the storm." I can't even imagine just what that tree has been through.
Flood, Freeze, and Hurricane, and much more, but that tree stands.
Let me explain what God said to me. He said, "Look at that one tree split into two separate parts. He said two trees as one!"
He said, "As Husband and Wife are also, these two are one." He said, "What he joins together, not what we have put together, what he has joined together it will endure until death!"
This tree and its partner will stand until death do them part.
Every day they greet the sun as it awakens the world.
Every night the moon brings peace as they stand before God together. Even in

their darkest time God still shines his light on them.
This tree represents true unity, two living things joined together by God.

—Dedicated to: Men and women, who have said their vows; they have been
   through the storm and still following God's word, unity.

These conversations always touch me. I'm a very emotional person. I feel and
relate well with my clients and allow myself to express great sympathy toward
them. My client hands me the poem back and asks me, do I sell my work? I tell
her she is more than welcome to it because God uses us through word, and the
places he puts us to be His helper. I know that God works in this salon. There has
never been any negativity in here. If I can't help you I sure won't hurt you. God
blessed me out of my sleep with this place. I had been looking for a place to rent
and kept being turned down due to a few credit situations. I told everybody
God's got a blessing for me; my little saying was "Crazy Faith"—faith so strong
it's crazy. I believe that's the faith God wants us to have, along with good works.
I believed, and one day God woke me up out of my sleep and said, "Go back to
that place on Old Spanish Trail. The lady is going to give you that salon. I followed the word and did as He said. My husband asked me where I was going and
I told him what God said, and I was obedient to the word. When I got there the
lady said "I was waiting on you to come back. If you want the place it's yours." I
had to tell her why I came back, that God had done it again. He said, "If you follow my word and have the faith of a mustard seed I will give you your heart's
desire!" People don't believe that faith with good work is powerful. So I know the
type of work God opened this place for, and it wasn't for no messy salon, but a
place for women to hear about what He has done for me! Don't get me wrong,
we had lots of good times in here, laughing, talking crazy, and on a good day we
even dance. I have a few clients who'll stay all day having fun with me. When
someone needs the word I give it to them. I don't go around all day preaching
that the body is like God's tool. If you have a hammer in your closet to use, that
doesn't mean you walk around with the hammer in your hand all day. No, you
know if you need it you can pull it out. That's how God is; He is in you, you're
his tool, and He will pull you out and use you if He needs you! Mrs. Johnson
really needs a warm word today. She is so full today with this problem, I just feel
for her. I know she can't go to a close friend with it. She definitely will think
twice before bringing it to a family member. These are problems you go to your
grave with, all to yourself. This is stuff family and friends never let go of and they
never let you forget. It's the reason we pretend life is so great, to stop others from

having a field day at home on the phone, e-mail, and whatever else they would do to pass on the conversation on.

As the old folks would say, "Getting it all behind backwards." By the time you hear it again it'll be so turned around. Child, you heard the Johnson's having some problems. "They say": we love those ugly words "They say," you know it ain't all the truth when they start with that. Another one of our famous sayings is "I don't like being in nobody's business." But then they say something so out of order just to spread something, even if they don't know if it's true or false. Gossiping just feels good and you know you shouldn't be doing it but its like a disease once you get it; you just have to tell somebody. That crazy "I'm just telling you, so don't you tell nobody I said it," well, if somebody told you and they asked you not to tell, what makes you think you can tell someone and they'll keep it to themselves? That's how negative news travels, leaving the poor victim worse off. Now you can't leave the house without people looking at you all funny. As if they don't have something going on in their life that needs their attention. In life your pain ain't so bad if you can spend your time talking about someone else's pain.

In my salon it's a different story. I don't repeat anything said in my salon to me, and my clients know this. That's why they are so comfortable telling me the real deal. For one thing, I don't know Mrs. Johnson, so she's free to open up, and the way I handle myself tells her she can take that chance. I began to do my thing; I pull out some of the things I've heard over the years from my grandmother and older women. I know it's hard loving a man who has fallen from grace. Someone you've loved for years, now you don't know these newfound ways and what triggered them in the first place. The mind is powerful and challenging; it will question you as a person you're holding a conversation with. Questions like: What happened? You thought you knew your husband, but maybe you didn't after all these years. Then Satan steps in with his questions: "Why are you allowing yourself, all that you stand for and believe in, to get taken away and devalued by some unhappy man who has lost himself and now chooses to have company in his misery by bringing you down with him?" That's how Satan works; these situations are opportunities for him. He steps in with all these negative mind games and it becomes war of the mind really. God wants you to come to him with trust and sincerity. Satan wants to bring hurt and pain, to break you down and make you lose your faith.

That war began the same way it did with Eve in the garden. God tells us, "He will lead you the same way he did Moses." Satan tells you, "If I was you I'd take everything he's got and leave him." See, Satan comes with destruction. God, on the other hand, already told you there would be some rough days, but he also told you that he was going to be there for you. It's like the teacher gives you a very hard test, so hard you hate the teacher, but she gives you a study guide before the test. Now, this test just makes you want to give up; you've come this far in class and now you get this test that just throws you for a loop. What do you do? The teacher is standing there, she in the class with you, but this is your test. Even though the class is full of people you feel so alone. You feel as though you're the only person in this situation, yet you see the teacher there and the other students and they are going through the same struggle.

Now after the test is taken and you've given it all you got, the teacher comes along and works a few of the problems out on the board. See, she waited first to see what you would do; after she gave you a chance to prove yourself she steps in. What a relief and how easy she made it. That's how God works. He is standing with you. You've got to prove you know Him and keep His word. God said, "My people parish from a lack of knowledge!" Not because they didn't have money or weren't good fighters but to know God and His purpose is where you gain life and all the blessings of life. Most of the time in a family the women have very strong faith in God. Men have always been told to handle their business. Now we are dealing with a problem where a man has run into a life lesson.

You know the old saying, "misery loves company." That's all this is. Satan has decided to use this brother; he has caused him to lose connection with his inner self. Confused, lost, he doesn't know how to ask for help or acknowledge there is a problem to his spouse, who is his helpmate. Satan takes these men and turns their life upside down until they don't know where to turn. These demons are out there on their job and they attack and destroy. My grandma used to say, "Keep your house prayed up." She used to say, "You a lie, devil, you gon' get out of her!" She would say, "I rebuke you Satan in the name of Jesus." She would demand that devil to get out of her house. Grandma use to say, "Be careful who you bring into your house. You don't know what kind of demons they're carrying into your home." She used to have saying for everything, but that's another one I believe in. Your home is a place you want full of good spirits, not those fussing demons or those distrusting demons. You have to keep prayer in your home!

Growing up, women are always taught to pray about a problem we may have. Men are taught he's a man and he's got to handle his business. This leaves the problem on the man, to carry his burden until he no longer handles it but is broken down by it. When a man is worn down it still may be hard for him to fall down to his knees and call on Jesus because of his tough-man mentality.

I tell my sweet client, "Look at her husband as if someone has invaded his body." I tell her, "You know the type of man your husband truly is. Something has brought him to this point in his life."

Ask yourself, were there any changes going on with him, settled ones you just ignored. A lot of times things happen to men, like jobs that make them feel disrespected, but they choose not to share with anyone. Men have told me that the race card is played in the workplace as a mental incapacity against minorities. The problem can become such a burden in some cases, and unspoken it eats at your manhood, causing some men to act out in strange ways.

There's also a ghost from the past that haunts men, things that went on in their childhood days that we have little control over. They try to carry on and lead a normal life but one day this problem comes knocking at their door. Without a strong spiritual background and without a true connection with God at the time this thing comes for you, you will find yourself lost, broken down and seeking relief in all the wrong places. See, the Bible speaks about being strong in the Lord. The reason is that we as humans in the flesh deal with a lot of carnal warfare: the battle of the mind, body, and spirit. These are constantly at war to find common ground for peace. God told Satan to go test his faithful servant, Job. Now some may wonder why God would put Job and anyone else through all that. See, the spirit and the flesh must testify to one God. As you are physically challenged in your everyday duties to be a good person, God comes along and gives you a deeper challenge, a spiritual challenge that everyone will see played out. He shows that through faith and believing in him you will come out a winner. Without a challenge, how can your faith in what you believe in be questioned? It's easy to stand before the church and quote those vowels. It's easy to love someone when it's all good. It's easy to say "my better half" when that better half's got it together, but what will you do when that other half is down. Like Donnie McClurkin says "We fall down but we get up!" Will you be there when he gets back up again?

As time passes by in a relationship things are revealed. To be able to still be by that person's side and say, "I know it's hard, but Baby I'm here" is like Job not cursing God. You take your partner and you bring that problem to God. He dusts you off and makes that stain on your relationship white again. He'll make the two of you His faithful servants in the eyes of everybody who thought they knew what the outcome was to be. The testimony that the two of you will give will make someone else say, "we can make it!" It'll keep someone from giving up on life, knowing that someone prayed their way through a serious situation. The Bible says, "Faith with good works prevail the righteous." Job never cursed God, he was used by God to show us that it gets hard but this is how to handle it. None of was used like Jesus Himself. Can you even imagine what it must have been for your father to send you out of heaven to be tortured for the sake of others? On this earth and in the flesh we will always be challenged, but you must always be prayed up. I tell Mrs. Johnson God loves her and wants her to love herself as well. God wants people to see the beauty He gave them, and they should respect it and know they hold great value.

Change is hard with anything you do for the first time: from riding on an airplane to having a marriage problem come into your life, it's hard. Unless you allow yourself to accept what's happening in your marriage, you go through your grieving period because you are human. Do whatever you feel like doing: pray, cry a little. Just because you pray that doesn't mean you can't cry. Now when you start the crazy talk, you know your prayers ain't helping. When you say, "I just feel like dying" and all that stuff, you know your faith is weak and you need a good prayer partner. Tell yourself you should be going through pain, that something great is about to happen in the midst of it all if you believe. Accept the death of the old relationship, a relationship that carries great memories of many wonderful times shared together. Pack it away—let those beautiful days be packed away into your heart and mind. Unfortunately, this packing away is part of your complete self to be put away, to move into your healing expecting to cry, and do all the things a person grieving goes through. Never give up on your healing at the end of it all!

During the end of anything there's always the feeling you get. It may not be a painful feeling like you get when something tragic happens but it's a feeling of closer. When you read a good book, that book is so good you hate to put it down. It comes to a peak; you sit up all night to find out what happens, then it's over! You don't want it to be over, than you wonder why it ended the way it did. There are no answers; it just did. Then there's all of the if, I bet, and so on. But it's over; you must close the book, put it away as memories. A life you once lived, a book you once read, they came to a peak. With the book, that's it; with marriage you become anew and much stronger in the Lord for healing.

7

When Reality Comes a Knocking

Not many men gonna do like Usher did when he told the girl in his song, "Everything that I've been doing is all bad." He says, "He got a chick on the side, and he been telling so many lies, He just gotta let her know." Like I said, not many men in relationships are gonna come out and tell you the things he's been up to. In return, you have to decide where do you go from there. I don't believe that bad things that going on in your marriage means that the marriage is over. I think the marriage you once knew is over. Another healthy relationship can develop through prayer and a lot of counseling, something both parties have to want.

Mrs. Johnson looks at me and says, "You make a lot of sense." She is glad she came in today and met someone who was able to handle such a conversation. I don't know her nor her husband, so I'm able to give advice that isn't one-sided. We as women need to be a little more passionate toward our sistas who are going through things in their marriage. That period in their life is so crucial: it's a moment when we feel like life is just not worth it! Marriage is something women feel defines who they are. It stands as a sign to the world that she's wanted, she's not alone. It's something society has put great value on. It's the one thing we feel we must do as women at least once, or you're made to feel less than a women, not wanted. A lot of our problems are passed on from one woman to the next generation. We as little girls are taught girls are angels. We are treated different from boys. We got more than boys—clothes, shoes—we were made to feel special because we were girls.

Little girls always played dress-up and put on a little of their mama's Vaseline to make their lips shine. You know, back then we didn't put lipstick on; people would say you was acting fast, trying to be grown before your time. Vaseline was the safe way to go. Mama would comb your hair to perfection, sometimes a little too tight but perfect. We played in Mama's shoes and her old dresses. We formed our own little fantasy world where everything is centered on us, the little girl;

that's what everybody told us. "Oh, she's so cute, you're going to have to watch her. She's so pretty the boys gonna go crazy." Only to find out in your little world this lie will only drive you crazy! For you and your beauty hold no value to this world and the worries that lie ahead. As a little girl you hear all this make-believe stuff and that's exactly what it is: make-believe. That's where sistas spirits still remain sometimes: in our make-believe world. For we have not yet allowed our womanhood to concur with our make-believe childhood! I hear all the time woman saying, "Well, you know my daddy gave me everything I wanted." Then she has to face reality: life doesn't give the woman everything she wants. This effect causes some breakdowns sometimes. You know: reality check. It ain't always the way the book said it would be!

We are sistas leaving the house with all the wrong baggage. Sometimes in life you have to leave a bag; its no longer needed in this lifetime. This sista sitting here is carrying one of her childhood bags; hopefully today, we'll clean out one. Dress-up she had down pat. Her hair was tossed up high on her head, real sexy looking. As if you pulled the right pin out, that hair is going to flow like a river. Her makeup was perfect, lips looking like cherry candy, glossy and perky, ready to be enjoyed at any minute! Eyes just the right shade of color, giving her a seductive look. Cheeks looking like red pillows, soft, and just the right amount of color to lift them up and make you want to cuddle up to them. Eyelashes that extend out from so much mascara, each lash looking like fingers, motioning "Come here, baby." Sadly at this moment her target is off a little. Mr. is not there to answer her call. With all that facial expression coming out, she looks like a sista ready for the world. Really she's just a scared little girl up in age. It's like being ready for war without a gun! You know what it's like to be looking in the mirror preparing for the day, trying to look your best, with all things in order, wanting to be adored by your mate. Wanting to be all he needs, desired by him. You are his queen, his lady. Everything your man desires, you want to be. She had the appearance down pat. The mind was not prepared—there she was empty. Brokenhearted, in a relationship that is killing her spirit.

Remember I spoke about the lady earlier called a strawberry, well this is one of the reasons she's in that position: beaten down mentally by people who were supposed to care for her, only to show her one day that it all was an illusion, causing a pain she could not handle along with other life letdowns. So never feel too above her; say a prayer for her. We come close ourselves to giving up daily. We deal with life issues that just hurt us. It may not be our husbands, it just may be that you're not where you feel you should be in life. Be real to yourself: it gets rough. I brush through this scared childlike woman's hair slowly, touching her with my warm, loving hands, knowing she needs my attention. Now that we are women we are not touched by loving, caring hands anymore. We tend to put up this strong woman image, when truly we need somebody to just wrap their arms around us and just say "Its okay!"

Let yourself be that soft little girl for a moment, allow yourself to just tap into her, love her for a moment. Let her just rest a moment. Oh, how tired she is. She's had to be a big girl all day long, dealing with life's issues; now just rest. Since we were alone I gave to her all that I could, my loving warmth that all little girls crave for. I'm all hers: no rush to finish her, since I see a sista in need. I allow her all the time she needs. For a moment we stare into the mirror just a moment. Her eyes show so much pain when I look into them; it's a pain no muscle relaxer or pain pill could cure! I think to myself, "This shine that people call bright eyes is just frozen tears that haven't fallen yet!" For she carries a cup full daily, waiting to overflow. I tell her, "Look at yourself. You are somebody who doesn't look at the face. Look deep into the mirror." Almost like we used to do when we were kids, looking deep into the mirror for Blood Mary, something kids made up to scare them to death. She looked at me to see if I was serious. I gave her that motherly look that said, it's okay, I'm here. She does what I say and the room becomes very quit. You couldn't hear a sound. Feeling the chemistry of pain mixed with disappointment, allowing it to be okay. It's okay to be feeling this way, it's the one way in the direction to making change. Just stare at her deep down within, looking into the window of your soul. You may get scared; fight the fear. Know that something is taking place for change in your life. Once you enter into your inside, just look at it! Feel how it's feeling and allow yourself to connect with that feeling. It's going to go like this!

Leaving The Pain Behind

When a heart has been in darkness it knows no place.
When a heart has been in darkness it can never grow.
This heart has been in darkness; it can never shine.
This heart has been in darkness and it does neither, for its muscles are so weak it causes a slow flow.
It whines as if rusty, it flutters as it beats, this heart is in darkness.
Damage has taken its place!
How can I leave this darkness and stop this pain?
For this heart has no life, nor does it wish to find one as long
As this heart's in darkness.
I can see the light, but can't seem to reach it!

Why am I stuck in this dark place?
My heart screams to just find peace, yet it's never delivered in any way.
I want to leave this darkness; yes Lord, I do!
I want to leave this darkness and find you!
You're all around me so close and near I want to feel you right here.

—Dedicated to: Lost souls

8

Stop Telling This Lie!

Taking this feeling in, let it touch your deep soul. This is where we get off track: it went like this! Well, well. So now I'm grown with my husband in the big world. The fairy tale went like this! Go to school and get yourself a good education. Then some young man gonna come along and sweep you off your feet. You're going to get married, move into a big house, start a family, and live happily ever after! Well, they lied to most of us. That story should stop being told. Yes, you go to school for that education: trust me, you're going to need it when you find yourself looking for a job. That young man, yeah, he'll come by looking for you and may marry you. The sweeping you off your feet you'd better enjoy, however long it lasts! Yes, he'll marry you, this beautiful woman that he just can't do without. This is before you move into the house that comes with bills, which means somebody's got to be on a *job*! Normally he'll do that, or the two of you will. The bills come so fast it looks like life picks up speed. Time is very important now. You don't have time to sit around smiling at one another. You use to be just a-blushing like you've seen a circus clown. Those days go, right along with the money to the bills. Having beautiful babies, yes they are special, but do they bring on a new and different world? Yes they do. If you thought life was challenging you, you haven't seen nothing yet! For as fast as your money goes to bills it goes to Pampers and milk!

Don't get me wrong; this is a great moment in life. You bring home this beautiful part of both of you. You just love it so much! But truth to the matter, it changes things! It's a financial adjustment that must be considered. A lot of you has to go to this bundle of joy. The two of you are now parents, responsible for this bundle, which brings on a different character that neither one of you ever met before marriage. You don't know how much of a change it's going to be. Trust me, it'll be some changes! It brings serious responsibilities that make you or break you, one or the other. It can make you into a loving family, working together, loving together, loving and sharing the responsibilities between the two.

Most of the time this is the way it goes, especially when you have very little support from family members, being there to give advice or physical support.

On the other hand, if you find no family support and it's just the two of you, it can get hard and confusing. The change seems to happen overnight and it's overwhelming. You begin to wonder, can you do this? Did you make a mistake? Bills are coming fast and now a new baby to adjust to. The home is totally consumed and now reality starts to set in. Now what? You either pull together as loving husband and wife or this is where the fairy tale ends! That Stevie Wonder song, "You are so beautiful to me, you're everything I need," that thought can start to fade away. The part where he says, "You're everything I need" ain't so true no mo'! My client is looking into the mirror and I can see she doesn't want to connect just yet. I say to her, "It's okay," knowing what I mean. A tear falls from her eyes and I tell her, "Let go, its okay, we all have something buried within us to let go of." I begin to tell her about the Lord and how he'll give her strength to deal with this.

Second Samuel talks about faith in God, believing that he will deliver you in your hard times as he did with David. David spoke to the Lord and he heard him, and delivered him from Saul. I tell her, "Unless you ask him to come into this situation, it'll only get worse." For God is not a rude God. He'll never just get into your warfare without an invitation; you have to ask him to come in. Like the old song says, "Jesus on the main line tell him what you want, you just call him up and tell him what you want." We can only carry so much before our foundation falls; it'll crumble, for our strength is built on emotions, which crumble easily. Jesus our Lord and savior is the foundation. He carries us all in the palm of his hand. He says, "Ye that are heavy burden." He wants to carry you through, but you must ask.

I again begin to witness to her about the Lord, for He is our comfort. He'll wrap his love around you and deliver you to peace. Tears just rolled down her face and I watched as the makeup flowed through the river of tears. I thought of the water baptism and how tears represent new birth, washing away the pain with each tear. Manifesting anew, thank you Jesus, let those tears flow, my sista. When they hit the floor step on them, binding Satan, taking back the power he thought he had. We don't realize what fear is, a sign we don't have Jesus with us. Jesus is strength, so in the name of Jesus say, "I bind you Satan in the name of Jesus!" Claim the spiritual healing and be blessed. God is a healer and Jesus is ready to lay hands on you if you ask him. This ain't no Keith Sweat or no Gerald Levert. These hands got *power,* baby! He don't need to rub you down, He don't need to touch your hair, He just needs to know you need him. He'll touch his child gently and a healing will take place! Jesus is a healer of your mind, body, and spirit, and relationships. Sometimes our relationship needs a healing and Jesus is right there. I finally realize what that song means: "Jesus on the main line, tell him what you want." Yes He is the main line. Any time you need Him, just say "Jesus" and believe in His name. He'll be right there!

The old folks used to hum that song all the time when I was a child. Now as a women I know for myself you need him every day, and ever hour. I say to her, "You and your husband are going to beat this!" I say to her, "I want you to go home pull out some pictures of happy moments you and your husband shared and lay them out throughout the house. Put one wherever you think he'll see the picture. Bring up a conversation about one of those pictures, laugh about it, and walk up to your husband and touch him. There is power in the touch of loving hand. Touch him and say, 'I still remember all your good. I still remember the way you used to make me laugh. You are still that dear friend and companion I married, regardless of any challenges we may have to concur!' Tell him that in your vows you spoke in front of God that you would be his wife for better or for worse. Don't challenge what you know is happening, you'll make him feel up against the wall, just nurture the wound without asking what happened."

Too many whys can cause a person to withdraw and shut down even to what is good. I said, "Tell your husband how proud he has always made you feel being his wife and how you want to keep that respect for him. Let him know it's going to be okay, whatever the problem may be, if he hasn't lost his love and respect for you, the two of you will walk through this. Still not saying what the problem is." See, when a person feels love and support from you before they feel judged, they are more likely to open up to their downfall without you bring it up to them. All that person knows is there is something you know, yet you show true love and understanding. Sometimes we do things and wish someone would stop our self-destruction for us. We must always remember, nobody's out to bring shame and unhappiness into their family. Through something very painful we can find ourselves doing things we would never have done otherwise. We must stay conscious. This person is not the problem; the problem is the invader that has interfered in this person's life, and they to wish it to end without judgment.

You know, I must say, when a piece of gold is found, it's deep down in the dirt. You take the time to wipe it off and bring the shine back. Now if you're one of the crazy ones you say, "Oh I'm not touching that dirty mess." You're too high and mighty to pick up a dirty blessing. I say dirty mess because a lot of treasures are found down in the dirt. Sometimes our life gets downright dirty and we feel worthless, but God sends the right person along to shine you back up. I say to

Mrs. Johnson, "Go home and shine your masterpiece of a man up. Today you do a little man dusting, dusting away yesterday's dirt and cleaning up the jewel you know God dropped down to you." Feeling no fear of rejection, this husband and wife can move out of this serious problem through love and God and moves on as a prime example of a today's Job.

My client hugs me and tells me I'm a godsend. We smile and pull ourselves together before my next client comes in. After it's all said and done, my lady looks good: hair is together and she's got a lot of positive thoughts flowing through her mind. We hug each other meeting as two strangers coming together for a service, ending with a bond of emotional healings, a bond as spiritual sistas that'll be forever. I bet today was a godsend for my sista. Tomorrow my sista will have a good morning.

9

A Word from the Therapist

Sisters, I hope out of this book we can find reasons to want to understand one another in a more passionate way. Knowing that we are just how the old folks say: "Overgrown kids at heart." We still like having our girlfriends to truly depend on. Smile more to one another. A smile causes the body to feel warm, it gives you that "it's okay" kind of feeling when someone smiles at you! Actually it adds life to you. It has been studied, emotions and what they do to the body. It is a known fact that a frown produces stress on the body, whereas smiling causes good health and a sound mind.

Let's make some changes in our lives, today as you read this book. No more accepting unhealthy relationships. No more looking at a sister like she did you something! In many ways we are connected. I love you all, my rainbow of sisters and I hope in my book you had an eye to see and an open mind to make some type of change in your life toward happiness. I hope out of this book comes understanding for all victims in this same situation. A husband who's lost and can't find his way and the two sisters caught in the sinful web of lust, confusion, and pain—just outright sins of this world that any of us can fall into. Never are we too above this world of spiritual and psychological warfare. It's a daily mission to stay together mentally and physically, praying for strength always.

On this journey I'm taking you on, allow your feelings to open up, and think hard. We all know someone who's going through something. After reading this book try something different. Go talk to that person who you know is going through something, not judging but actually being there to listen, praying to yourself as you listen to the person speaking. This very act is going to make you feel so good and a blessing will be waiting for the two of you afterward.

Independent Woman

What a great day! The sun's shining, the breeze feels great. Lets see what I'll do today. See, I'm an Independent Women, I take care of myself! I answer to no one. I worked hard to get in a position to take care of myself and control my destination. Yes, yah see me, it's like that. So today what shall I do? I know what I want: to have a great day! I start by having a hot bath to soothe my body. The water felt great, temperature just as I wanted it, nice and hot, bubbles to praise my skin as I slide in. What an aroma to tickle my nose—the sweet smell of gardenias prancing around in my head. I got comfortable and closed my eyes, saying to myself, "There's nothing like starting the day off just as I please, cause I'm an Independent Woman!"

The room's so quiet, so perfectly set, as if I prepared it for a guest, One sure came! There was no one standing there for me to describe. No one there that I could scream, "get out!" to. This is my house! No one there to say, "Do you know who you're talking to? Yet the invader began enjoying my pampered moment. It just took over without getting any say-so from the Independent Woman. That energy took over and I cried! I was not in control. I was not capable of running the show at that moment. See, it was the mind of the Independent Woman, all that this invader brought without an invitation. It didn't respect that I was in control. It had no respect for how I planned my day. So today I realize to be independent is to stand tall, look strong, smile as you may, but know that there is a mind up there you don't want to mess with! Just as you plan that perfect day it decides it wants to deal with some hidden things, the Independent Woman begins to cry. So am I Independent or what?

—Dedicated to: All the hard working sistas who have cried during those crazy days, just when you thought you had it going on!

PART II
Let's Talk About the Said-to-Be "Good Old Days"

10

At the Beautician

Oh God, don't let it continue to rain. Not on Saturday morning. Black folks ain't coming out in no rain to get their hair done.

It's seven o'clock in morning. I got up early to beat the rest of the family so that I can have some quiet time for myself. I always say one day God is going to bless me with my very own room, so I can close the door and everybody will know that's my space, and when I'm in there it means Leave Me Alone! Like Oprah says, "Create a little spot for yourself, put candles everywhere, giving off the perfect aroma of something sweet and pretty. My favorite flower to smell is the gardenia.

Recently, I got the chance to smell the best room spray. It was a pumpkin spray. That spray smelled so good, I swear I was ready to eat. So no, I can't have that spray. Lord knows I cry every day to lose a few pounds, so, I guess I'd have to stick with the flower spray and candles.

I have this picture of a beautiful lady, lounging on her front porch. The setting is a beautiful Acadian house with a wraparound porch built on the bayou, with the most beautiful lilac-colored wisteria flowers hanging from the trees. Along with the flowers, moss hangs from the old trees. She sits in a beautiful white rocking chair with her legs up and crossed on the rail of the porch. The bright color on the painting looks as if the sun is shining down on the world with pride as it delivers the completeness to this beautiful day.

As I look at that picture each day and I say to myself, "The God I serve is going to bless me to one day. I'll find that peace I see this lady possesses and that joy she seems to be reflecting and that welcoming spirit of calmness I see across her face. She looks as if this is how Eve would have been in the Garden: carefree and right at home, one with nature.

I hear someone go to the restroom and it snaps me out of my desire into reality again. Lord, please let that person go back to sleep. I enjoy my mornings. It's when I'm most inspired to pray or just be one with myself before going to the shop and having to serve everyone.

Oh Lord, a loud thunder shook the house and lighting shone through the window. My goodness, this is truly a rough morning. I tell you what it makes you think of: the power God has.

Lights are flickering off and on; I see we're gonna lose power in a minute. Good thing it's morning time. Here comes the poor dog, Queen, looking at me like "What the heck is going on? Somebody better pick me up." I bend down and pick up my daughter's little Chihuahua, my little grand puppy, and cuddle the poor thing in my arms. She's just as bad as the kids 'cause now I got to fight off the kissing and the climbing all over you so. There goes my morning.

Well Lord, every day is a good day. Even these wet and gray days are of you, Lord, and I thank you. For without the rain, we could not appreciate the sunshine. So Lord, I thank you.

I look outside and the trees look as if they're having a rain dance party. They are rocking to the tune of the thunder and the leaves are going with the rhythm of the wind. I say, Lord I have seen a heavenly form of salsa. Looks like those trees was doing more shaking than Jennifer Lopez when her hips are at their best. It didn't top this dance performance I was watching. Made me want to put that dog down and start shaking somethin' myself. I said, "Girl, go sit down!" Ain't many imaginations like mine. I just find life in everything God gives us. He gives good weather for the humans, bright sunshine, wind blowing. Just enough to make you want to let your window down in your car and just drive. Let's say when the Democrats are in office and we can afford the gas.

See, when President Bill Clinton was in office you could ride in yo' big SUV. Now Bush is in office, you have to let yo' windows down while you go and come from work 'cause gas is so high now. I don't care how pretty the day is, once you are home from work you don't leave for no joy ride. Unless you live in a city like New Orleans; you can get on the street car and ride. But not after Hurricane Katrina, and how long the government is taking to rebuild New Orleans back up, you don't have that to do. Again them Republicans, for the good old boys as usual. As we know, New Orleans ain't no good old boy city.

This day, and the rain that it brings, is a joyous day, for it delivers to mother earth all the nourishment provided by the Almighty. Through the rain comes life, washing away all the old, leaving the earth fresh and new. After a good hard rain, the sunshine's so bright, the leaves on the plants look beautiful and green. The flowers spring up nice and pretty. So as you watch the rain come down, know that it is delivering life. Can I get a what? Thank you, Jesus.

Somebody needs to wake me up and distract me from myself; in here lettin' my thoughts get the best of me. I need to be gettin' dress for work, but you know black folks don't move around much when the weather is bad. We was always told to get somewhere, and as Ma'Dear say, "sat down somewhere." Them black grandmas meant just that. Playing while the Lord was doing his work was a quick butt whooping. Taking a bath during bad weather was out of the question for black folks. We was told if you was in some water and lightning struck you, you could get electrocuted and die. So, you know what that means … I ain't gettin' in no water this morning.

I'm scared to take my gown off 'cause you know what they say: "If you don't have yo' shirt on when its lightning, you might get hit." Lord, I'm a be late today: can't bathe, can't take yo' shirt off. All you can do is like Ma'Dear say: "Sat down" before the Lord knock you down while he doing his work.

Well, I have a little time to wait before getting dressed for work, so me and Queen find us a comfortable spot to sit and chill. Queen lies down and I close my eyes for a minute: another thing that was taught to us as children was to sit down and pray while the Lord did his work. Before I knew it the time had passed, the weather looked better, and it was safe enough for me to move around without getting' struck by lightning.

11

Slippin' and Slidin' My Way to the Car

I look into the mirror one mo' time before I dash to my car.

As I'm trying to walk out the door, I hear my son asking what he's gon' eat. You know, I don't know who these old experienced teenagers are these days, thinking you were just put here to serve them. He'd better make an egg sandwich and get his butt up and do some weekend cleaning. My daughter says, "Ma, can I come get my hair fixed today?" I say, "Lord, I don't know what they gon' do when you bless me to take as many trips away from here." I've done my job. I don't have no mo' little babies to take care of. I scream back to my daughter, "Girl, don't come to that shop all late. I'm not playing with you."

Baby, I stepped out that door and slipped down in some mud and slid almost under my car. I started talking to myself: "Now look at this mess." Them doggone children done worried me till I done came out here and slipped almost under my doggone car.

You immediately think about who saw you. I looked around by the neighbor's house to see if somebody saw this mess. Please, in the name of Jesus, don't let nobody see me down here on this nasty, muddy ground. If you ever had a chance to see how my daughter and I walk, you would know why I wouldn't want nobody to see me on that ground. For some reason, we have this twist that makes women roll their eyes at us, or they'll say, "I knew that was your daughter by the way she walks." I'm thinking, how am I gonna walk into the house without them sickening kids asking me what happened to me. They'll see all this mud but still ask something crazy just to make me answer them.

I get on up, look around, and carefully walk my wet behind into the house. Of course, everybody's still in bed. I could have been dead, and they wouldn't find me until later that afternoon. Thank God my weave didn't get wet with this mud. Lord knows, I hate to redo this hair.

I run into the hall bathroom to get out of those wet clothes, hop into the shower real quick, washing away my morning adventure. I bust out laughing. I know the rest of this day has got to be better. I get out the shower and, by now, my husband is up. As I come out of the bathroom, he's looking at me like, "What are you doing up in there?" Then he looks down and sees my wet clothes and he start laughing, at the same time asking if I'm all right. Yeah, its funny, I must admit—a hell of a way to start your morning, slipping your behind down. He takes my wet clothes for me and puts them into the washing machine while I get dressed. Go ahead and laugh; I don't mind. Laugh your way to that washing machine, my good hubby.

Okay, let's try this again, walk my behind outside again. This time, I'm taking my sweet time, twisting with respect to the wet ground. I got into that car and drove off into my day of adventure at the beauty shop. With a beginning like today, this is going to be one heck of day. Make plenty money and have some good laughs while making it.

At the red light, one of my clients is in front of me. It's funny, 'cause whenever a client sees me, they always look into the mirror to see what their hair looks like. So she sees me and automatically looks into her rearview mirror. That just tickles me every time someone does that. I be thinking, girl, don't worry about your head. I'm over here looking like my hair done been through Hurricane Katrina all over again. I toot my horn at her, letting her know I ain't acting funny. You know we can trip if you don't speak. It'll mess my little cliental up. You better always have an eye for your clients. Call it a third eye if you want, but you better speak if you see them. Our people is somethin'. Next thing you'll know, that client will be sitting in somebody else's chair 'cause you was tripping and didn't speak to them when they saw you passing by. Now did you hear me? When they saw you passing by. Now, maybe you didn't see them and evidently they saw you. The smart thing would have been for them to say hi to you, since they did see you first. No, honey, that would be, as my grandma said, too much like right. No, let's make some drama out of this. Oh, she's acting funny. The beginning of something you know nothing about! That's the truth. I ain't making that up. You better have three eyes or else!

We pull off from the light and she toots her horn. Which means we're straight for the day. Looks like the sun's trying to peek through the clouds. Oh come on, sun, so these folks can come out to this shop. Nothing like a long, slow day at the salon, waiting on folks to drift in. Oh shoot! What are they doing up there? Working on the doggone road. I know we have to make room for growth, but I hate sitting in traffic. Only one side is open on this street so we take turns letting one side at a time go. I think things would move a lot better if brother got off that doggone cell phone. I know it ain't his boss 'cause he's smiling too much. I want to scream so bad: "Get off the doggone phone and do your job!"

Since I had my little adventure I'm not feeling so all that quiet yet. So I sit here and wait on this fool. Ooh finally, doggone it, he lets our side go. My li'l client turns. Oh well, she ain't headed to the shop, at least not mine. She's straight; I'll see my girl soon, I'm sho'. I'm wondering, since my morning was so crazy, who my first client is. I need a good laugh to cheer me up, so I'm hoping it's someone with some humor this morning. I can use a little "No girl, you crazy" right about now!

12

Yes 'N Deed

Oh yeah, I see my girl. It's on now. Just who I need to pick up my morning. Tammy's sitting in her car waiting so she can get the heck away from here. First, before she leaves, I know she's got some crazy stuff going on in her world. Sista is an Internet freak. This girl know she be doing some stuff on that Internet. I tell her all the time, "Girl, you gonna get yo' butt caught up! Keep on with your crazy self."

I blow my horn at Tammy before I pull into the parking lot. Let me run in and get things started since we're the only ones here right now, due to the bad weather. Our people don't like to get out of bed when its raining. That's one reason there's so many li'l colored children. Rainy days make love. Between the rhythm of the rain as it crashes down on the roof of the house, it causes couples to want to do a lay-down dance to the wonderful sound of nature. Nine months later, you wish you would have found something else to do besides stay in that bed.

Tammy ask, "Where's everybody at today?" I look at her like, "Now, you know yo' people." We laugh. Girl, look, you better come on here and enjoy this moment. She says "Yeah, but I had a bone to pick with ya'girl Stacy." "What happened?" I ask. Tammy says, "Girl, that heffa told me to come to Dillard's Friday; she would be able to get me on part time. I go looking for this cow and she ain't nowhere to be found. Wasted my morning. I'm waiting to hear what lie she's gonna come up with. You know I can get the job on my own, but she said the person that does the hiring and setting up your days since. I'm in school, I don't want certain days. So, Stacy said she would talk to the lady since they are sorority sisters. I'm looking all over for her."

"Girl, I can't wait to talk about that wench," I say. "Ooh, Lord girl! She done upset you. Child, maybe something came up. You know Stacy got yo' back." Tammy say, "Yeah, that heffa knows how to have yo' back when she needs something. I ain't heard from her since Friday." I say to myself, "Yes, you are getting a quick "do" today 'cause I don't want no drama up in here this morning. I done fell down, slipped all the way to my car, had to go change clothes, business slow due to the rain … so I don't feel like listening to no sista arguing about no job and who was wrong."

Colored folks can do some arguing over nothing. I don't know what part of Africa or slavery it comes from, but it definitely needs to go back. We can ruin a beautiful moment with some crazy mess. Don't try to plan yo' day around our people. Lord, somebody's gon' trip! That word, you remember, can get ugly.

"Girl, come on let me get you started," I say to Tammy. "When was the last time I relaxed yo' hair? We need a little help with mother nature's effect on a sista's head today." "Look, don't look at that situation the way you're looking at it. Girl, God got that, trust me. What's for you, he has already put your name on it. He knows exactly how you want it done and he has worked it out. Now, when you do get this position, you owe no one gratitude. It's a blessing between you and God, so release it, girl. Look I'm-a go back here and get this relaxer. I'll be right back. You think about what I just said. If a client comes in while I'm in the back, tell them to make themselves welcome, have a seat, I'll be back."

As I'm walking to the back, I say a quick prayer: "Lord let thy will be done, Lord, when it comes to that job." We humans believe all we got to do is want something. We don't ask God if our wants are of Him! We just want it now. Think about it. Example, how many times do you just have to have a particular dish? You could just taste it. What do we say? "Ooh, I can just taste me some barbeque chicken." You walk around all day long talking about that barbeque chicken and how bad you want it. We so crazy, we tell the Lord, "Oh Lord I can taste me some barbeque chicken." You get on the phone and you tell yo' girl-friend, "Girl, I have a taste for some barbeque chicken. If I get a chance, girl, I'm-a make some 'cause I just got to have it, or I'm-a go crazy." You know, we say all kinds of crazy stuff all day long. Well guess what? You spoke on that chicken. You done prayed, "Oh Lord," you done everything possible to tell yourself you need that barbeque chicken. You finally get up Sunday morning. You gon' throw down: barbeque chicken, potato salad, and some green beans with garlic bread. "Oh Lord, I finally got my barbeque chicken and stuff." You sit down and eat like you done lost yo' mind. Three hours later, you got heartburn, yo' stomach hurts, you just don't feel good. Your night is all messed up. Now you got to take something 'cause you done ate that doggone barbeque chicken. Look in the medicine cabinet: nothing for upset stomach, nothing for heartburn. I be, doggone, I ain't got nothing in here so I can go to sleep shut. Lord, I don't feel like gettin' dressed to go to no Walgreen's. Okay now, you done got yo' prayers answered 'cause you wasn't satisfied until you got yo' barbeque chicken. Now, that you've eaten this meal that you just had to have, or you was going to go crazy without, you praying to God 'cause it made you sick.

What I'm trying to say is, even though this is a small example compared to some of the things we put into our minds that we need, we don't always pray for what is good for us. We have to learn how to look at things sometimes before asking for it because it looks good, or someone else has it and it looks good for them. That job may have looked perfect from the outside. The hours, even the pay, but God knows what goes on in the inside. Maybe He didn't feel that was best for you at this time. It also can be a situation where things work out for the better for you when you approach the situation on your own.

See, you never know a person completely. You know one side or maybe two but we, as humans in the flesh, we carry many, many faces and there may be one you haven't seen. But they have on that job and you wouldn't want that person to speak for you anyway, so God stopped it and wouldn't let it be. Sometimes we just need to thank Him, no questions asked. Just "Thank you Lord, for you stayed ahead of me, and you worked it out." Even when we feel this is it, guess what, just maybe it was it, but not for you. Alright Lord, You in the house!

I thought I was gonna get my laugh on. Oh no, Tammy gonna be Tammy this morning. We not gonna do this old depressing crap. I get my relaxer and walk back into the salon area. I ask Tammy what kind of trouble she's been getting into on that doggone computer. Tammy comes up with some stuff, I tell ya'.

One time Tammy found this guy on the Internet and they seemed to get along great—always had something to laugh about. They had the best conversations together for hours at a time. So you know how it goes. The day comes when it's time to meet. They decide instead of him coming to Slidell, she would come to New Orleans. That way, she knows she won't have to worry about him being on her turf. This guy's name was Terrance. She said his pictures were really nice and made him look very attractive. He had the looks sistas approve of, someone you can be seen with during the daytime—you know how it is. So, Tammy came in, got her li'l "do." You know I hooked the hair up for my girl. She was straight when she left. I set her hair, then put her under the dryer for an hour. Once she was dry, I wrapped her hair around her head and placed her back under the dryer. Sista's hair was bouncy, full of body, and very pretty when she left. Just the way you want it to get your flirt on. Toss the hair a little bit, turn your head, let it flow with the rhythm of your lust. I told her "Girl, work that hair." Men love them some hair. Why, I don't know, but if a sista got pretty hair, I think it just makes a man trip. Ugly as death, but pretty hair: it's going down … brotha all in it.

When Tammy got up out of the chair, she looked in the mirror, did her li'l dance we do when we think we're cute. She shook her hair like she was Tyra Banks or somebody. I said, "Work it, girl, work it. Now lay some money on a sista!" Tammy know I was clowning. We always cut up. Since she thinks she cute, she says, "Girl, I ain't got no money," I say, "Well you ain't going on no date today; get the broom and start cleaning." Tammy says, "Oh no, I'm going meet this fine man!" She pays me and heads out the door as a car is pulling into the parking lot. "All right chick, don't do nothing I wouldn't do," I tell her as she leaves. Looks like two more cars are pulling up all right. Lord, this is what I'm talking about; let's make some money up in here.

"Hey girl! Come on in. What's up? Long time, no see. Where you been hiding? I haven't seen you in a while."

"No, girl, I've been sick lately and wasn't feeling up to getting out. I haven't worked all month. My doctor took me off my job and told me to take care of myself or else. So the take care of myself won."

"Oh Sharon, I'm so sorry to hear that. Girl, I tell ya. You just don't know. Girl, you should have called me. I would have came over to wash and grease you scalp and keep your head feeling good, you know that. Girl, get you a seat. What you doing today? Is it relaxer time?"

"Oh yeah—girl, this hair is rough right about now."

"Sit in my chair, Sharon. I'm-aa get my girl back to her old self."

"Girl, that old cancer is back. Soon you won't have to worry about no perm. Doctor is going to start me on my chemotherapy treatment. Which means the hair will be going again."

"Well Sharon, look. One thing we know is you have strong genes 'cause that hair sho' came back after your last treatment years ago. We gonna keep the faith that God got this too. In the mean time, we gonna make you look and feel good today."

"You know Mr. Mark died."

"Oh no, I didn't know that"

"Yes, he's gone on to glory, child."

"Well, you know Sharon, he lived a good life. He was a daddy to all the children in the neighborhood. I remember when we was little kids, my grandma would send us to the store to get a few things until she went into town. Grandma knew all the prices to everything. She would give you just enough to make her purchase and she never went over with too much money. Grandma had counted tax and all into her total. Mr. Mack was the store owner, and Mr. Mark would say "Mattie sent you to the store, didn't she?" and we would all laugh. There would never be any change to buy candy with either. Mr. Mack would give you a free piece of candy or Mr. Mark would buy you something while he was in the store. He would always ask if you been good in school. If you said yes then he would give it to you. I know a lot of kids is going to miss Mr. Mark."

"So have they set up his service yet?" Sharon said.

"Not yet."

She was sure we would know something soon since all his family made it into town. Man that was one great man. We will miss him.

"So, Sharon you're hanging in there, I know. We gonna do as we did last time: pray you through this too."

"Girl, look, I done been there, done this, and ain't gonna let it get me. Thank God for all of the pretty wigs. When the time comes, I'll just get me one, have you cut it to fit me, and strut my stuff."

"Girl, I hope when I'm faced with something as serious as this, I can keep a positive head like you. You just amaze me; I think about how you hold on so strong through it all. Sharon, I'm thinking maybe we can go ahead and cut your hair into a short style. That way as your hair begins to shed, it won't be so drastic. Girl, look into this new book I have with these cute short cuts. Girl, these styles are sure to make a man do whatever it is that makes twins. You know what I mean? Make a husband throw-down girl, ya' know?"

"Well, girl, if you think its gonna do all that, then give it ta' me, baby! Let's do this!"

"Hey Trishia! What's up, girl, take you a seat. I ain't gonna be all day. Let me get Mrs. Sharon going, then I'll be ready to get you in my chair."

"Girl, take yo' time. I ain't in no hurry. I'm away from that house and ain't in nobody's rush to get back home to them buggers. Girl, I look forward to this place. I know I'm-a get my mind right," explained Trishia.

Trishia talks to Sharon. "Good morning," as usual. You know we must speak to each other and keep the peace, colored folks. They began a conversation, catching up on old news. Trishia brings up Mr. Mark. "Such a sweet guy," we all say. Well, I hope that church he belongs to is large enough for his guests, 'cause we gonna be there to see him off to heaven.

I comb through Sharon's hair, which has grown out to her shoulders nice and thick. I tell ya', some people just have good genes. Okay girl, here we go, I take all the back and cut it off completely. One … two … three … it's gone. Trishia looked like, "Girl, you done cut all yo' hair, as pretty as it was?" Trishia asks, "Now why did you cut your pretty hair off?"

Sharon says, "It's just hair, baby. I ain't worried about it."

Little did Trishia know Sharon was getting' ready for a good fight, a fight for her life, and she was being a soldier about it. Nobody would have ever thought Sharon was going through all that she was, not from the way she handled things.

We all laugh when we think about the time people spend putting weave in and here she was cuttin' hers off. That's how life is, isn't it? The "haves" and the "have nots." You have it, most of the time you cut it. You don't have it, guess what, you buy it. No biggie. The problem is, nobody wants to be behind the have nots, and the weave job that's like a horror story. The end result beautiful.

"So did ya'll sleep good this morning when all that rain came down?" Sharon said.

"Look, after Hurricane Katrina and all that I went through, I don't sleep good when that rain is coming down like that. I got up, looked out my back door to see how those trees was looking, since we're still waiting on the guy to come cut those trees down."

"Girl, I don't know. It's just different now. You know, growing up here in Louisiana, we get rain all the time, but now that we have gone through a horrible experience like Katrina, baby, I respect the weather."

"I was not just going to lay in that bed while that wind was whippping up out there. I got on up. Got me a good ole' book and got into my book," said Sharon.

"Girl, what you reading?" I asked.

"Girl, I missed ya'll so much over here, I went out and bought this book called Salon Therapist, volume one. Girl, when I tell ya', that book is something. I hate to put it down."

I ask her what she think about it. Sharon says, "Girl, I have been by myself reading that book and laughing like I'm in the room with other people."

Trishia said, "You know, I keep saying I'm-a go buy that book."

Sharon said, "Well, girl, go buy it. It'll make you look at your stylist different. It allows you to see far beyond a hairstylist. I love my stylist, girl. I just never realized how much more the salon is to us."

"Well, I've got to make my way over to get that book," says Trishia. "Sharon, you're looking good already and your style is not finished. I hope I don't have to call that man of yours and tell him he better meet you in the ladies' room 'cause you gonna be straight."

"Yeah, right. Funny. That doggone man is a mess. No telling what he's doing at home, pulling out of that shed he done built to put away all his things. I tell you that man have some tools and man stuff. I think he needs everything he sees in Home Depot. I guess he do work hard.

I tell her, "Girl, long as he brings home the bacon along with all them tools, it's all good. Just don't look at him and his mess."

Trishia says, "Girl, look, don't talk about yo' husband. Baby, some of these old, sorry men don't know what a hammer is. They don't try to do the things a man's supposed to do and know to keep things going. Girl, look, these old, sorry boys trying to be just as cute as the girls now. You go into the nail shop, they're in there gettin' their nails done. So that tells ya' he ain't doing nothing hard with his hands."

Sharon says, "Yeah, that's true. All these Diddy wannabes. Now you can't tell the man hands from the woman. It's sad what television is doing to this generation. I think some of these rappers have sold their souls to the Devil for the almighty dollar. Nowadays, to describe what the role of a man is, you'd have to find a book to describe it to you 'cause you don't see many young brothers coming into that manhood."

Trishia says, "You know, girl, now the woman is the strong one in the household. She keeps the family going while these young boys play dress-u" and entertain their friends with the thought of them pimping their way into success. It has really gotten sad."

You know money is the root of all evil. What people won't do to have it.

Coming up, we were taught to respect each other. We were taught to strive respectfully for success and make your community proud of you. Now, it's strive for that dollar, selling your soul and everything else to achieve it. And guess what? It's working. I remember hearing someone say when I was a little girl that the end-times were going to get so hard that the only people who would have money were those who had sold their souls to the Devil. I'm sorry to say, but I think we are living in those days. The things our young brothers are doing to make a dollar, it's so sad. They are prostituting their minds and their bodies for riches. We are seeing a generation destroyed as we did during slavery. It will take years to heal this direction we, as black people, have allowed the media to bring into our homes, schools. Our community, which we once prided ourselves on, is now like a sewer. Garbage is being delivered daily, cuttin' away at the beauty we once knew.

Sharon says, "Girl, what happen to the songs you was proud to be singin' 'cause it made everybody want to sing it and feel good about themselves? Two sistas riding in the car sing that James Brown song "Say It Loud—I'm Black and

I'm Proud." What happened to that song, "Fire-Ya"? Oh no, the "Funky Chicken." You know those days, everything meant something respectful."

"Girl, some of these songs, you wouldn't want nobody to hear you sing them and when you do catch yourself singing them you have to question yo'self. I know I'm not singing that song. Check yourself, as they say. We all laugh, 'cause it is something that we all find ourselves doing sometimes.

"Girl, I know at our li'l career day in our black communities, our poor black kids just know they want to become a rapper or a ball player. I wish I had a way to take kids out of the 'hood and expose them to other areas in life," said Sharon.

You know, when my kids were little, I would drive them around and show them houses we could not afford. Then I would tell them to pick out their house in that area and every now and then we would drive over to see their house. That was one of our Sunday drives out of the 'hood into my children's future. All things are possible through faith and good work if you just be determined and strong. My kids love to drive and look at what they could have. I never wanted my kids to feel like they could only live in the black low-income communities just because we were there at that time. Believe you me, Mama and Daddy hadn't given up their dream three kids later, and guess what: we got out. My kids were raised in a middle-class environment, went to good schools, and lived a life their parents never knew. They saw two determined parents who were not giving up. No, we didn't get to Turtle Creek, but we didn't stay in the 'hood either. Thank you, Jesus, for hearing my prayers 'cause that's how we made it. I talk to the Lord. I told the Lord I had to raise my kids in a good environment, in one house. I couldn't be moving my kids all around Slidell. I told him what I wanted and through faith and good works we got it and still live a good life. God is good if you trust in him. Baby, when God blessed me with my first house, I shouted so loud, my husband thought I was looking at something on *Oprah*. What I was doing was praising God.

Girl, now that I'm thinking about it, you know God does things so funny sometimes. God puts you flat on yo' behind, then He'll raise you up. He says, "Come all that are heavily burdened." Bring your burdens to him. You know I was dropping off some burdens at that time. Look, it was like going to the laundrymat: drop it off, pick it up once it's done. You know, the Lord keeps his word. We are just some crazy "right now" people. Faith is a form of waiting and believing. You know, we're so crazy. Ask somebody to do something for you and see how you feel when they don't do it when you felt like they should. Our first remark is "Don't worry about it, I'll do it myself" or "I thought you was going to do such or such." We just can't wait, it has to be done to satisfy that person right then when we ask, or they will get quick to say something negative about you. That's us: "right now" people.

"Sharon, look at you, girl, we done talked you right into a new look and girl, you are ready to go now! Brother man gonna check up on it!" Sharon stands up and looks in the mirror, does her li'l dance. You know when we feel good, us colored folks like to dance. Sharon does her li'l dance; now she's feeling good and ready to get in trouble. That man gonna wanna know where she thinks she's going, looking so tight.

"Now, girl, put yo' lipstick on and you straight," I say.

Trishia says, "Now hook me up just like that but leave me a little length in the back. You know my ancestors are with me. Even when I get a relaxer, my little be-bes still wanna curl up in the back, so leave me some hair that I can curl with a small curlin' iron."

"Girl, you is crazy, but I know what you mean; sometimes my little be-bes wanna jump up from under my weave. That's when I know it's time, baby, to do my redo. Can't have no bad weave job. Oh no, walking around here like some of these poor sistas. I just want to pull out a chair wherever I'm at and say, "Baby sit down, let me help you 'cause this ain't it. Almost, but ya' not there yet."

Trishia's laughing so hard. She says, "Girl, you are crazy. I swear, that's why I don't mind coming and waiting. I know I'm-a get my therapy up in here."

Sharon says, "Well, I hate to leave ya'll good folks, but I got to let the world see my stylist's work.

I tell her "Go on girl, show that head."

"Ya'll a mess."

"Come on, Trish. Let me get you going. Girl, this rain, this morning made colored folks lazy. That's how them surprise babies pop up. Sistas better get out of that bed and come on in here before they get something a little more than a hairstyle." We laugh 'cause we know it's true. A rainy morning makes some good lovin'. Just look at all these Hurricane Katrina babies. Girl, them women should have got out of that bed. No stove, make that husband build a fire. Girl, move around, do something. Have a ham roast with the fire. You know somebody had some Vienna sausage. We always buy them for bad weather. Have a camp out, whatever, just get out of that bed before everybody know what you and yo' husband did when the lights went out. We gonna mess with ya' you know that.

"Oh look, we talked ol' Sonya up. I know she gonna be glad ain't many people in here. She hate to come when I'm busy." Sonya gets out the car, twisting like she's on a runway. I always tease her about the way she walks. She gonna cause a wreck in front my shop one day. The men be just-a blowing and acting up. I guess I shouldn't complain; at least she has on clothes today.

"Hey, y'all. What's up with this weather? Child, I thought I was going to be stuck out today. Girl, you know I'm going to that Maze concert tonight."

"Oh ya, I forgot about that with all this bad weather going on. Girl, that's going to be nice, the kind of music grown folks listen to, music you can dance to, get your grove on to, wave yo' hands in the air to the sweet rhythm of soul baby." "That's what I'm talking about," we all say. "Now that's music."

"Girl, you know you wasn't gonna let no rain keep you from gettin' that head together, not my girl. Sista hooked up all the time. You ain't gettin' ready to mess up that rep," I told her.

"Girl, look, I was praying that rain let up. You know I was nervous."

"Well you know I gotcha!"

I thought about going to this concert, but we all went to the last one a couple of months ago when he came and the Commodores came to replace Teena Marie. We enjoyed ourselves at that concert. It hit the spot to see a crowd of colored folks enjoying music without degrading one another, causing hostility in the audience. With Maze, you can sing the song and enjoy yourself. The Commodores played their song "Fire." We jammed to that and I hated where we sat 'cause, on the floor, people was gettin' down.

I think that's the kind of fun God would want us to have: good ol' clean fun. Music that brings out the happiness and good within us, you know, not this crazy music you're hearing blasting from cars nowadays.

"Sonya, I know you not going alone, so who's the lucky one tonight?"

Sonya said, "Ya'll ain't gonna believe this. I was in the Quarters last month and girl, this fine-as-wine man came up to me. Girl, I can't tell you just how good this man looks. Girl, he must have been first in all God's beauty lines. He had a body that God must have molded him himself. It look like it took all six days of the week to make him and everybody had to rest on the seventh."

I said, "Sonya, you don't have nobody's sense, girl. I just don't know about you."

"Girl, wait! You ain't heard nothing yet. This man walked up to me and looked into my eyes and said, 'Hello, my name is Derrick. I find you very attractive and would be pleased if you would enjoy the remaining of your time with me!' Girl, I was lost for words and you know I'm never lost for nothing. Baby, that man has me just lost. So anyway, girl, the man put his arm around my waist before I could say anything. Well, I guess the look we both shared, the way we both was breathing, as if we just ran a marathon and needed water dashed on us

… okay, not water to drink, girl. No, we needed to be brought back to earth. So I finally got to the point where I could say something. Softly, I said 'Well, my name is Sonya and I find you just as attractive and would be pleased to enjoy the evening with you.' My mind started talking to me, girl. I was like 'Shut up mind, quit tripping, leave me alone, please; for once, listen.' Oh no, girl, my mind was telling me 'girl, do you smell him?' Lord, this man brings weakness to your body. The aroma from the sweetness of his body mixed with the sexiest cologne. I think the man was dragging me cause I know my legs were not cooperating with this body at all.

"Girl, he looked at me and asked if I was okay. I tried to be cool and give off a small, girlish smile and say 'I'm fine' and my doggone voice cracked. I said, Lord please help me to be able to enjoy this creature that you let walk the face of the earth; and he walked his self right onto my path. Girl, I never prayed so much. My girlfriend managed to whisper 'ol' heffa' in my ear, girl, but look, I didn't care. I acted like she was saying something just as cute. I giggled all cute and she looked at me with eyes that made me just want to holla. You know how crazy we get. The night went fine. We talked, got to know a few things about each other, and we have been seeing each other ever since. Girl, I can't believe I'm acting like this 'cause you know me; I pimp them niggas. I know most of them ain't trying to help a sista, so I don't treat them like I need them but to entertain me, then 'to the left!' This guy Derrick calls and asks if I'm all right, do I need anything. Girl, at the beginning of the month he asked me for a deposit slip so that wherever he's at with his job, he can make sure I'm straight to take care of myself until he gets back. I was speechless. That was something that has never, ever happened to me: a man stepping up to the plate. I said 'Lord, I don't know why this man is in my life or where we will wind up at, but Lord, I thank you. You have shown me that true men exist. This man has never tried to disrespect me in no way. He walked into my life and he has been nothing but a blessing to me.

"Girl, I'm just another Sonya. We talked about all the hurt I've been through and trying to make it in these streets alone. Girl, look, we went there about everything I've struggled through. I just felt like he was the one that I could open up to about myself. I told him about my early childhood, the sexual abuse from the men in the family and close friends of the family who knew that my parents was never home and was able to walk into our unprotected home and use me as they would a common whore. I hate to call them by that term, but you know society gives everybody a title and a level of respect or disrespect through that definition. Girl, I know ya'll know my people so it ain't no secret to what happen to me and my poor sista. You know, look like God always put someone in your life to help you heal through past pains, someone who loves me for me. Someone who knew no one in this town and could care less about what other people feels. You know, I always believed in God," Sonya said. "I just always wondered when he was going to give me a break."

"One day, I remember just like it was yesterday. It was a Friday and I didn't go to school that day. Nobody was home to wake me up for school and nobody was there to get me ready. You know, as black folk, we have to get that hair comb at least every other day. Well, this Friday, the hair had been pushed to its limit so I woke up feeling lost to the world and no one to say 'Good morning' to. No one there to ask if I was hungry or did I sleep good. Just me and my little sista. Poor Ebony; she looked up to me. I did all that I could do to protect my little sista. She was all I had, all I knew. I would wake up to her in the mornings, and we would hold onto each other at night when we was alone.

"This Friday was, as usual, the beginning of the weekend partying for the adults in the family. They went to the local bars and left the kids at home to fend for themselves. Unfortunately, we couldn't always do that and so the party began like this: the first male adult that got drunk and came to our open house came to two scared little girls who just wanted to go to sleep and drown out their nightly fears of being alone. This night, I remember so well, a friend of the family came home smelling like old cigarettes and alcohol: a smell I'll never forget. He stumbled into the room the two of us shared. As we held onto each other for dear life, not knowing which drunk this was entering into our room of horror to be the inflictor of this terror. I had no choice but to push my little sister to the wall and deal with this nightmare in the flesh. I prayed for God to let this be the last time anything like this happens to us. Lord, I don't know why this happens to us. I don't know what we could be doing wrong to get punished like this, but Lord, when I find out, I'm-a quit doing it, Lord, so you won't punish us like this again.

"You know back in the days, ol' folks use to say 'God gonna punish you if you lie,' or for whatever reason they choose to tell you that lie! That night I got raped at least twice by this man who used to come over all the time and play cards with the family. I fought as hard as I could, I took my nails and tried to scratch him up, I bit him as deep as I could. I didn't want to scream 'cause I knew my scared little sister was in that other room and she had no way of helping me. I didn't want to scare her any more than what she was already going through. The smell from this man will stay with me for the rest of my life along with the damage he and everyone else caused that used me. I went back into the room with Ebony and held her close to me, hoping my little sister would believe all this was just a dream: that we could wake up for the next day. The next day would take care of itself because when you came out of the bedroom into the living area you would be reminded that the horror you experienced was oh so true, 'cause there, laying deep in his sin, was the monster who destroyed all your beliefs in good nights. Those words never came out of your mouth, never knowing what your nights would be like. You never wasted those sweet words."

Leaving the Pain Behind

When a heart has been in darkness it knows no place.
When a heart has been in darkness it can never grow.
When a heart has been in darkness it can never shine.
This heart has been in darkness and it does neither for its muscles are so weak it causes a slow flow. It whines as if rusty, it flutters as it beat, this heart is in darkness and damage has taken its place. How can it leave this darkness and find a place. How can I leave this darkness and stop this pain, for this heart has no life, nor wish to find one, as long as this heart is in darkness.
I can see the light but can't seem to reach it.
Why am I so stuck in this dark place?
My heart screams to just find peace, yet it never deliver, in any way. I want to leave this darkness, yes Lord I do. I want to leave this darkness and find you.
Your all around me so close and near I want to feel you right here.

—Dedicated to: Lost Souls

13

Reasons We Have Beauty Salons

"Sonya, you know God sees all that we go through. He knows the pain we feel. As the tears are formed in your head to be delivered into the windows of your soul, God knows before they slide down the likeness of him, your face. God knows. He said 'suffer little children,' so he knew we would suffer as He did but He said 'come unto him.' He put the invitation out there for us 'cause he knew there would be days when we had to question life and the mystery therein. Girl, sounds like God is starting to work on you. He has sent you a helper as he did with Moses. He sent Aaron to speak for him. Seems like God has sent you this fellow to be a soother to your mind, body, and spirit." That's what I told Sonya.

"See, God knew from the beginning, when you were in the warm protection of your mother's womb; he knew that born into this difficult world would be a child named Sonya. He knew that there would be many trials and tribulations for this girl child. He, as his Father in heaven knew the pain this innocent child would face. He counted up the tears that would form inside your heart and deliver the message of pain to the brain and cause a rainfall of many tears to wash away whatever caused the pain. He knew each drop. He also knew the day and the hour that he would dry those tears up. He knew, as the last one fell, this day, my child, you would carry this burden no more. He said today is the day that I will dry up these waterfalls of pain, that he would cease all that had caused His child Sonya to hurt. As He's the one to cease the winds in the time of storm, baby: He ceased those tears. He gave you a story that will be with you forever to tell without shame, to let people see that he'll carry you through."

Satan You Thought You Got Me

There was a time when I was down: Satan you thought you got me!
There was a time I had to sell my body to feed my kids: Satan you thought you got me!
There was a time I had to steal to put clothes on my kids back: Satan you thought

80

you got me!
There was a time I took any man just to have one: Satan you thought you got me.
There was a time when doing drugs was the only thing to relieve me:
Satan you thought you got me!
But one day, something step into this body, and it began to move.
I began to cry, my body got full.
I began to shout, cause my body got busy.
I began to say, Thank you Lord, for I was delivered.
I began to say Satan, you a lie! I was found from the wickedness of this world:
Satan you thought you got me!

—Dedicated to: All the people in this world who have been in this situation and
are now delivered!

Trishia brings us back to the salon, cause child, sometimes this place gets so emotional somebody's got to break up the thick air.

"Stop, before I get full up in here and get my shout-on! Give me some tissue. Ya'll got me over here just done got plum ugly. If ya'll don't stop up in here … Girl, God brings up some conversations in the shop. Ya'll know what this is: our salon therapist. She knows how to flow for God. I'll tell anybody, you dealing with something go get yo' hair done by my girl. But for now on I'm-a tell 'em 'I know a therapist and she style yo' hair as she help you deal with that burden.'"

"Trishia, girl, you a mess. Let me get back to yo' hair; you gonna be in here with us."

"Girl, you know how I am, I just got to spread the word up in here 'cause you know what a blessing it is to share a good word. We hear enough sistas talking bad about one another and not sharing enough love. Ya'll know it's about healing and an understanding of the next level up in here."

"Sonya, girl, it's your time. Girl, look, enjoy it and don't, I said don't, let *nobody* steal your joy."

Trisha said, "Baby please stay focused. Don't let that ol' devil come into what you got going on. Even when you get nervous, say a quick prayer. Don't run away from what could be real with this fellow if he's doing what he should. Just pray and ask God to be in the midst."

"Okay Miss, hold this head up right. Now, you done started preaching. We is some preaching folks up in here." I told Trishia.

"Girl, you know I hold a bad head. My mama used to pop me with the comb. She said I ain't never hold my head the way she wanted me to. Mama use to say, she had the worst backache from combing my hair, so I guess I haven't changed that.

"Well, no Miss Trish, you haven't."

"Aah, Miss Therapist, leave me alone before I have to eat that pecan candy I got in the car for you," Trishia teased.

"Now, see? Indian giver. You brought it for me so you have to give it to me now!" I insisted.

"No, I don't. I haven't put it in yo' hands yet. I didn't want to bring it in and not have enough for everybody so I said I'd just leave it in the car and you can come out and get it and put it into your car. Now, if you gon' talk about my bad head, I'm-a eat my candy."

"Okay, you got me. I want my candy. Me and Sonya gonna eat that while I do her hair! All right, let me break my back as yo' poor sweet mama did, to keep a girl cute."

"That's right, hook a sista up. My husband might feel something romantic once he look at me, and start acting like Sonya's man. He just might have to wrap his arms around me and hold me tight." Trishia giggled.

"Go on, girl! Work it! That's right, don't hate; join the game baby, join the game. That's how that goes. Work it, baby!"

"That man, that man," Sonya said, "girl, he smell so good, when he walked up to me smelling like heaven on the men side, my legs got weak; I had to talk to myself. I said, heffa you better not fall out now. I said mouth, you better not say one doggone word wrong. I said eyes, you better not roll like something crazy. I said hands, don't grab that man!"

"Girl, you don't have no sense," we both had to say.

Sonya said, "No, if ya'll would have been in my shoes, ya'll would have had to get it together too. Ya'll know I can get ghetto occasionally. 'Excuse me, who you lookin' fa', all up in a sista's face?' But this was different. He was so sweet, he was kind and not all arrogant. He almost made me feel like he humbled himself to make sure I wasn't offended in any way as he approached me. I just don't know. The man makes me nervous. Sometimes my legs just get weak, my hands start shaking. I just don't know."

Trishia said to Sonya, "Sonya, if you don't think you can handle him, wrap him up and put him in the freeza' for my next life."

We fell out. "Yes indeed, y'all ain't right."

I Want You

Lurking into your mind I shall, only because I want you.
Lurking into your soul, digging as deep as you allow me, only because I want you!
Lurking past as your eyes observe the figure passing with plans of concur, only because I want you!
Lurking into the right moment when our mind, body, and spirit meet without words, but feelings of notice, only because I want you!
Lurking right into your arms, the place I long to be, feeling the rhythm of your heart beating tellin' me you want me after all, only because you want me!
I want you!

—Dedicated to: Love

"Ok, Missy, I'm finished breaking my back on you, so what'cha think, mama?"

"All right, now I ain't responsible for the night 'cause, girl, you done hooked a sista up. I done got my shout on and head hooked up. What more can I ask for. Oh yeah, I also think I've found the man to chase after in my next life."

"And just who that might be?"

"Sonya's new man: I'm sending up my prayers tonight."

"Lord, if I come back to this ol' world, please Jesus, send him on down right along with me 'cause Sonya describe a hell of a brother, and Lord, you know we all need a hot sexy brother to drive use mad sometimes. Lord, not that I'm not grateful for my dear husband, I am. Just next time, I want to smell this man who makes yo' knees weak. I want to have a reason to say, 'I can't go to work today.' See, my crazy self be done sat up and watched the man all night just wondering what was his mud mixed with when God made him. It sounds like a special dust, 'cause it ain't many of them in these neck of the woods."

We had no choice but to laugh at this crazy girl: "Girl, get out my chair and go home to Mister!"

Trishia got up and we hugged 'cause we all have shared something so emotional in here today. Yes, the rain kept a lot of the clients in today, but only God knows why he caused things to fall in line the way he did.

"All right, sista, you go on now and shake what ya' got so that man of yours can take you out to dinner; you and them youngins."

"Now, why you brought them up? Baby, they gonna stay their butts home tonight. I feel a little young and sexy. Mama and Daddy gonna go do somethin' tonight. You know, a little sum-sum. Then maybe we'll come home and I'll let him check up on me!" said Trishia.

"Get out of here Trishia. You are crazy, girl, but hey, I ain't mad at ya'. Beyoncé yo' self out of here.

Trishia leaves, and as she walks to her car I hear a horn blow. I look up to see it's a man blowing his horn. I stick my head out of the door and tell her she's already got somebody wanting to check up on it, so she know she working with a li'l sum-sum!

I walk back to my chair and Sonya comes and sits down. I place a cape on her and we discuss her "do" for the evening; since the weather's bad, maybe she'll want an up do. We look at a few pictures. You know this ain't the same ol' Sonya. Sista getting' her 'I'm the lady' look on now. Forget about that Shanaynay look, this girl got plans, baby. She is working on somethin'.

"So, girl, what us gon' do with you? Sonya, I'm so happy to see you so happy. You know I remember all that you went through. I always said it was sad you and your sister couldn't have lived with a better family member until your parents got it together. But look at a sista now. You are a beautiful girl and things is on the positive now for you, and we gonna give this to God to nurture into something wonderful. If anybody deserves to be happy, it is you. In life, we all need a break from Satan and all his works. He inflicts pain to break you down to curse God. He goes throughout this world testing God's children's faith through painful experiences. But God says if you can just trust Him and be ye faithful, He'll bring you through. So Sonya, he didn't bring you this far to leave a sista. He brought you this far 'cause now He is getting ready to elevate you to your next level. Jesus said 'don't worry about what people do to you.' He said he would deliver you in the presence of those who persecute you. All I want to see you do is hold yo' head up high and know that God is working it out.

14

Release and Be Blessed

Sonya turned to me and grabbed my hand. She looked up at me and a beautiful but painful tear fell from her eye.

"Girl, I'm terrified. I've never had anybody treat me this way. I tell myself I deserve him, then it's as if my mind is torturing me because it comes right back with, 'How can you deserve a man like this when you have been taken by so many men? How can you deserve this when you have given yourself to so many men?' I fight it with my own answers that I know are so true: that I never wanted this life. Many nights I cried myself to sleep 'cause there was no way out. There was nowhere to run, only to the place I never was protected in." Sonya said all this as she wept.

"Release it baby, release it right in here with me. We are alone and I'm-a put this closed sign up 'cause today we gonna get this devil out the way, so that you can truly move on."

I walked over and turned the closed sign on. I didn't want anybody to come into the salon when I could see that today God was ready to deliver someone that I had watched grow up in pure pain. I had listened to people talk about her as if they forgot what she had been though. How could a child be brought up to not have respect for herself through continuously being abused, then grow up to be anything other than confused and self-abusive? Her life reflected her past, not who she wished to be, but who life taught. I wanted to listen to my dear friend today without being disturbed.

I said, "Girl, we gonna close these blinds make sho' nobody come over."

Sonya sat there crying as I closed up. It had become so emotional for her to rehash this ol' stuff. She asked me, did I remember when her sister took her own life. Girl, my heart just got full and I took Sonya into my arms and just held onto my friend as she broke down and cried. Yes, I did remember. She just couldn't go on abusing herself the way she was. She just never found happiness and people always judged her wherever she went. She just got tired and gave up.

Sonya said to me, "There was just nothing else I could do for her, once she let those drugs take control of her pain. We lost her before she went onto the next level. It would be days before I would find my sister. Girl, I would be so sick just worrying about her. Then she would pop up from nowhere: hair not combed, needing a bath. I would run her some bath water and undress my sister and give her a good bath. We would sing the old songs we used to sing when we was kids as I bathed my sister like she was a child. I would use my special Victoria's Secret body bath in the water and the bathroom would smell so good. Then I would sponge my sister's back with the warm water. I just wanted her to know how special she was to me, regardless of what had happened to us and how she was dealing with it. To me, she was all I had. I would dry my sister off, rub her down with the best lotion, and dress her in my clothes. I'd wash her hair and braid it up for her so that it would last until I saw her again. My sister was dear to me. I swear she was; she was all I had. Lord, she was all I had." Sonya began to scream. "Lord she was all I had! Why, Lord? Why, Lord, Why?"

"Let it out Sonya, let it out." I just started praying as she screamed and cried. "In the name of Jesus, Lord have your way in this salon today, God. Lord, I said if you would bless me to have this place I would serve you in here. And Lord, today, we need you, Jesus. Lord, we need a healing of a wounded soul and a broken heart. Lord, mend this heart and seal this soul. Lord, we need you right now as this sista releases this heavy burden. Lord I ask that you deliver her."

Sonya got out the chair and dropped down to her knees. She let out a scream that brought chills to my body. "Lord, Lord," she said. "Oh Lord, what did we do to live the way we did? Lord, why'd my sister had to leave the way she did? Lord, why'd my sister never have a chance on this earth to live a happy life? What could she have done, Lord, to deserve that?"

The shop was filled with a spirit. It was a sad, broken-down spirit, shackled down from many years of hurt and pain inflicted by a world of lust, drugs, and just plain ol' sin. These kids were born into a living hell, known only to those who have gone through it: a life full of mental and physical abuse.

I say to Sonya, "God's got a plan for you, Sonya. He's working on you right now. I want you to just start thanking Him; right now, thank him."

We both started giving praise right there in that shop. We thanked God for what he was about to do for Sonya. We were thanking him for this great breakthrough. I said, "If we can drop it like it's hot, we can praise God without shame. Right now, we ain't got no room to be in shame. We were dealing with something neither one of us had any control over today. This was the day He chose to deliver this child of His. He designed this shop in His likeness. All I was was a witness to His deliverance and grace. We began to clap our hands and give praise. You could feel the spirit change from pain to rejoicing. You could feel God in this place. He said, "where two are more join in My name, I'll be there." God was in this place. These two sistas had prayed Him in. Sonya was up on her feet giving great praise, for she knew God was there this day to make a change in her life. He had given her a good man to show her that God created, just for her, someone special. This was what she needed to show her that she to could be loved without sexual contact, but with a strong mind and respect for her and her body. We prayed that He would lead Sonya, that he would show her how to be a good lady: that he would open up her heart and allow someone to come into the brick circle she built around her for defense. That if this was the right guy, He would bring them together to worship Him in harmony.

Sit Still

I can't sit still, you talk too much!
I can't sit still, you tell the truth!
I can't sit still, and you know why.
They say be still and let him do his work.
I can't be still, and you know why!
Deep, deep within there's this voice. It talks to me when I sit still and listen to what it says.
I want to cry for the words it says.
I know you know; you've sat still yourself.
The truth it says just that way.
It never sugar coats, nor softens its message: just the truth when you sit still.
Sit Still
The room so quiet yet so much is being said.
It makes you face what you wish was dead.
It says to you all that is true, cover your ears, close your eyes, scream out loud, yet the message comes and you can't sit still.
I sit here and let you attack. What words you choose to speak, forces that go so deep. Words never spoken to me that way. But the truth it is I must say, it's all the hurt I try to run from, you seem to taunt me in every way. I'm-a sit still and let you do this. Go ahead have it your way. See my legs are tired of running; what else can I do not to sit still. So I'll just listen and face the message that is determined to be developed.
Maybe he's working on me, but first I must sit still!

So what!
Sit Still!

—Dedicated to: All those who don't know who you are. May this deep thought
make you go within and find you.

Lord we command these words in your son, Jesus' name. Now, Sonya baby, let it
go. Let it go, right now. Baby girl, go now and live your life. What has happened
here today in this beauty salon is something wonderful. God has washed away
your yesterday and made your today brand new. He has come in here and washed
away the dirt. You may have felt used, but it prepared you to be His witness that
He is real.

Sonya got up and sat back down in the chair and we hugged again. I gave her
a big smile and asked her what it feels like to be cleansed by God. No caressing
soap, no Victoria's Secret, just the warmth He wraps around you in the spirit.
The way you feel when He releases you, there ain't a hot bath like it.

Sonya pulls herself together. While she's doing that I go into the back room
and give God my own thanks, 'cause I have witnessed Him again in my salon
delivering someone else out of shackles. Thank you, Lord. I know this is not a
church, but Lord you walked up in here 'cause my door is open to you. I gave this
salon to you the moment the key was placed into my hand. You have moved
around up in here on a many of occasions and I thank you. Thank you Jesus!

I walk back into the front area. I look at Sonya and she looks as if she is glowing. I tell her, "Girl, they won't be ready for this, Sonya. Beyoncé ain't got nothing on what I'm looking at. You gonna make that man hold your hand all night!"

We both laughed 'cause we know it's true. God has given her a new disposi-
tion.

"So how we gonna hook this hair up for tonight?" I ask.

Sonya looks in the mirror and runs her manicured hands through her head.
"Well I think I want it up. What you think? Something that won't look too bad
if it starts back raining? You know, I ain't ready to let this man see me look rough
yet; don't want to scare him off."

"Girl, please, this pretty head of hair you got!"

Hold My Hand

Hold my hand tickling my inside.
Hold my hand claiming me with pride.
Hold my hand as we parade through the city, saying many things without one

word.
Hold my hand claiming togetherness!
Hold My Hand

"Well, all I got to say is, look out Jay-Z and Beyoncé, here comes the new couple of the night!"

"Girl, I hope it be all that for a long time, not just tonight, cause this man is doing something to me."

"Well, long as the something is good, then let him keep doing it," I reassure her.

"Girl, let me turn this open sign back on and open these blinds up so folks can come up in here to see the new Mrs. Sonya!"

"Girl, stop!" says Sonya, blushing.

"Sonya, I ain't playing, girl. You is it now, go on, girl. I ain't hatin', do you, baby. Everybody has a season in life. Today, and the rest of your days, is going to be beautiful.

Season's Change

When the mind of a child turns into the mind of a young adult,
Seasons Change.
When the mind of a young adult turn into a Man or Woman,
Seasons Change.
When the mind of an adult develop away from the thoughts of yesterday,
Seasons Change.
To know your transition and where you stand in the midst of it, with a true
understanding of this Life Revolution is to know,
Seasons Change.
From your Transitional Journey from child to adult let your extended time here
on God's planet of manifestation show that through this journey of everlasting
lessons you was able to handle,
Seasons Change.

—Dedicated to: Everybody searching

"I want the world to notice you, girl. You have just had a breakthrough. You know how many people waiting on a breakthrough? Baby, you are blessed in your right-now time and your tomorrow; we claiming that!"

I walk back over to Sonya and we go to the shampoo bowl. As we're walking a car pulls up. I say, "See, girl? Here comes somebody. They coming to see the new Sonya.

Sonya says "Girl, stop!"

At the shampoo bowl, Sonya sits down, leans back, and as she's looking up at me, she says, "Thank you."

I bend down and kiss my sista on the forehead and say, "We in this life cycle together. Each time somebody come up in here and I can be of some help, I feel a blessing coming."

The door opens. It's a new client coming in.

"Hello, how may I help you?"

The young lady comes in with a little girl. She wants to have the child's hair pressed and her hair relaxed. I tell her give me a few minutes and I'll be right with them. I tell them they're welcome to have a seat and look at some books. It's nice to see new people walk into the salon; a fresh face just in time to see my new Sonya.

I say to Sonya, "I guess every little black girl knows about that pressing torture from generation to generation."

"Girl, I know. I remember my Aunt used to press me and my sista's hair when she would take us to church with her. Lord, that was the worst part of gettin' beautiful. It was times I felt like 'just let me look ugly.'"

We both laugh, 'cause that is so true to all of us. Until you saw a boy at church you liked, then you took that burning, to go to church smelling like burnt hair, but you was cute: shining like a new penny. Grease everywhere, enough to shine yo' face, arms, and legs, but we was cute!

"Come on, Sonya, let me put you under this dryer for a few minutes, to get most of this water out. You with all that pretty hair, I'd be all day blow-drying it," I tease.

I walk over and introduce myself to my new clients. Then we go over to my chair so that I could find out what type of relaxer she had been getting, how often she got them, and also to feel the texture of her hair to give my own opinion of what I thought would be good for her hair. She had very thick hair, shoulder length with a few gray streaks in the hairline. She had never applied any color to her hair. I asked her what was her plans for the gray; was she planning on letting them grow out or was she interested in a rinse today with her relaxer? She asked what I thought. She was only in her thirties and didn't want to start looking older than her husband, yet. I recommended, with her hair being so dark, she go with a dark brown, which would make her gray look like highlights. Then later, if she liked it, she could go with a permanent medium brown. Nothing too drastic, just enough to lighten her up a few shades.

Karen, my new client, thought that was a good idea. I went into the back to get my relaxer and start. I always start on another client while I have a client under the dryer: time is money in this field. Boy, if I charged for all the other stuff that goes on in here, I could sit down in between clients. I section Karen's hair off and start applying her relaxer and two more cars pull up. Horns start blowing and I hear somebody holla, "Hey, girl!" I don't know which car they're screaming at. This is how the beauty shop goes, lots of action inside, and if you're on a main street, you get a lot of action outside. I tell Sonya, "That look like yo' girl, Monica. She gonna talk about you. You got here before she did."

"Oh yeah, that's her."

"Is she going to the concert tonight with y'all?"

Sonya answered, "Now you know I can't go nowhere without her! She going along with her friend; this dude she been kicking it with for a while now. We introduced him to Derrick one night, going to the movies; they seem cool, you know."

Monica walked into the salon, "Hey ya'll! How ya'll doing." We all speak back, then she looks under the dryer and sees Sonya.

"Why you didn't call and tell a friend you was coming to the shop this morning, heffa?" she asks.

"Sonya says, "Now you know you hard to wake up in the morning. Then it was raining too. Baby I drug myself out the bed to get her so I can be cute for my baby!"

"Oh Lord!" Monica teases. "Ya'll should see her. She would have ya'll wondering just who that is, 'cause' baby, she act totally different when her and Mr. Derrick is together. She act all shy, like she can't talk. I be like 'Sonya if you don't quit!' But they are so good together. I'm happy for my girl, even though she didn't wake me up! Derrick is a sweet guy and he shows my girl true love. D, girl, they be so into each other you have to find a mirror to remind yo' self you with them. Girl, he is so sweet to my friend. I think she did it this time."

These two are so crazy they make my new client smile at them. I know she know how it is in a salon, so we bring her into the laughter.

Monica asks me, "D, you think I have time to run and get my nails done down the street?"

"Oh go ahead. I still have to do li'l mama over there and finish "Mrs. In Love" over there," I insist.

"Yall stop hatin," Sonya shouts from under the dryer.

I asked Monica did she know the car that pulled up with her. I didn't know. It looked like a sign on the door of the driver's side.

"D, I didn't pay any attention to it, I was busy gettin' in here."

A young girl got out with roses in her hand. We all jumped like "Okay, who gettin' them pretty flowers on this rainy day?"

The young girl walked in and said, "Hello, do you have a Sonya here getting her hair done?" We all turned to Sonya like, "oh no he didn't."

"Girl, what have you done to that man?" we say in shock.

Sonya's eyes got big as they could get and she started to cry.

I said, "Oh stop it and take those doggone flowers, Miss Special; read the card."

The young girl walked out after she gave the flowers to Sonya. I went behind her and gave her five dollars as a tip. She walked out so fast. I guess the child felt we was too excited to remember to tip. That I will remember, 'cause I like them too.

"Sonya, read the card. Hurry up, read the card. Stop crying, girl, and read the card."

Sonya reads, "Sonya, I knew you would be at the salon today and it was a wet morning. I wanted you to know even during the rainy days, I'll love you if you let me, Derrick."

We all was crying by the time she finished that letter. "Oh girl, what is he made of, special ashes? Did God give him some special dirt of the earth? Lord, I want one."

"Me too!" Monica said.

My new client said, "There's nothing like a beauty salon; everything goes. You never know whether you'll be laughing until tears come down yo' face or you'll be crying from something so touching, but it's all good. I love coming to the shop."

I work on my client and I just feel so good this morning for Sonya. Life is amazing, if you can just hang on until your time comes. It's time for this young lady; it's her time!

Monica gives Sonya a hug and says she'll be back. She places the flowers on the table for Sonya, then she leaves. The shop has such a happy spirit in it. I love these days when the unexpected happens in here.

"Karen, I think it's time to rinse you, baby. Come on back here with me and I'll get you rinsed out." I tell her daughter she can come to the back if she wants, but she's content with the cartoons on television.

"Karen I'm-a deep condition yo' hair, then I'm-a put the rinse in, then we'll go from there. While Karen's hair is conditioning, I'll take Miss "In Love" from under the dryer and get started blow-drying her hair completely dry so that I can flat iron it once I put the rinse in Karen's hair. Gotta work it. That's the only way you gon' make it.

Sonya sits in my chair and asks me, "What am I going to do?"

I say, "Enjoy it and let him show you what a lady is supposed to be treated like. In return, you treat him with the appreciation that a woman shows a good man. God put him there for a reason and he'll work it out. Just do the right thing and enjoy. Shit, I ain't got no flowers delivered to me while I was having my hair done."

"D, it's so good to talk to you. You know there is no way I could afford to pay you for all the therapy I get when I'm in here. Girl, you should change your name to a salon therapist, because a lot of times when I leave you I feel so refreshed."

"All right, y'all gonna make me up these prices including all my therapy I give out," I teased.

"Girl, wait until I get my ring and some I-do's going on, ya' hear? 'Cause a sista be stretching it sometimes. But baby if I get this man, it's all good. I'll be able to hook a sista up a lot better!"

"Girl, look like brother-man likes what he sees, so do what you supposed to and the brother gonna be there.

"Sonya, I'm-a pull yo' hair up in the back, then I'm-a swoop the bangs and pin curl the top. It'll hold in a little rain. You'll still be cute if that happen."

"Sound good to me baby, I know you got a sista; so have at it, do yo' thang."

"I hope the weather stays all right the rest of the day. Nothing like gettin' wet in yo' nice outfit."

"Girl, yes! 'Cause I went out and bought me something nice, but eye catching, you know. Not too revealing, but enough to get a brother wondering."

"Alright Miss Thang. Girl, look, I'm learning. I'm gettin' there slowly. Sonya, remember nobody changes overnight, so always be grateful. God has brought to your attention a desire to change. I'm so happy for you. You just don't know how happy."

"D, I know if anybody wish me well, you're one of them. Thank you girl, thank you."

"All right, girl. Close your eyes, here comes the last of all this hair spray to make sure you keep this cute look all night: rain, shine, or some good, strong hugs. This hair will last."

"Ooh Girl! This is cute. I like this a lot. This is going to work for me." Sonya stands up a does a little happy spin, checking herself out.

"Yes ma'am tonight bro-man gonna be checking up on you. I know when he sees you along with that cute outfit, you gonna blow him away."

"D, I just want this to last forever. I feel like a little girl with a crush on a classmate. He makes me feel all tingly all inside!"

"You and yo' tingles! Have fun now. Go get yo' self together. This style's on the house. I'm happy, you happy. Now out! Go get yo' nails done. Oh, and don't forget those beautiful flowers. I'd love to claim them, but you deserve them and all the good that is headed your way, my sis!"

"See you, D. Thanks Girl. I'm gone. Bye ya'll."

As Sonya walks out of the salon, I can see a new woman. The way she walks: so sure of the woman she is, a proud strut to her walk. A walk not needing the approval of no one. The way she is dressed today is much more respectful to her. She is so beautiful. That girl is gonna make it, I do believe.

"Karen, I'm-a rinse your conditioner out in a minute. Let me get some juice for your sweet little girl and also mix up a color. I'll run back here real quick."

"Lexus, do you want some juice, baby? I have those juice packs. Would you like one?"

"Yes, Mama, I would like one please."

"Now that child is raised. You don't just get those manners off the streets. Mrs. Karen, you doing a good job with Miss Lexus. She is so sweet."

I walk into the back room and realize it's nice to come in contact with a well-mannered child. She has been sitting down since she got here; she hasn't been all over spinning in my chairs like somebody with no upbringing. This child is wonderful. Thank you, Lord.

"Here sweetie. I hope you like fruit punch. That's all I have left after my big kids come here and drink up everything."

"Thank you, ma'am,"

"I just love this child. Can I take her home to show my grown kids what they was suppose to be like?" I chuckle.

"Go ahead, you can have her. She'll talk you to death, then you'll bring her back." Karen jokes.

"Oh yeah, I know those little girls can do some talking. I have one myself and yes she can talk when she is in the mood. Come on, Karen, let me apply this color to your hair. It's a reddish brown that'll look warm on your skin. Then we'll pull a few strands through the cap and give you a few highlights."

"Girl, I'm-a be ready to go to the mall and show off my new look. I can't wait until it's done."

"That's right, go get me some business. I'm-a make sure you turn heads, which will make sistas ask 'who did yo' hair?' So, I'll make sure you have a few of my cards."

"Girl, today has been one of those days. I knew it wouldn't be that busy with the weather the way it is today. This is one of those pull-out-the-ponytail days. One of those go-into-the-closet-and-pull-out-yo'-best-friend, whichever one go with the outfit. That ol' wig; it never fails ya'."

Now sistas it comes a time in life, you have to depart from these friends. You have to send them to "hair glory." I know you hate to spend money but the wig must go after a while. I hate to see a lovely sista with a tore-up wig. Baby, get a new friend 'cause' that friend is no longer your friend. She got you all jacked up. Let her go. Close yo' eyes as you throw the wiggly little friend out. Have somebody take the trash out of the house to make sure you don't go get the dead friend. She is gone.

Now, those ponytails; I swear I hate they sell them without instructions on how to wear them. Okay, here we go. Here's a little ponytail lesson. Number one: if the front of your hair is thin do not, I said do not, go out and buy no long thick ponytail and stick that thing on your head. That ain't cute. That ponytail should be no longer than ten inches and you should take it to someone to fit it on your head. It should be thinned out as much as possible to make it look as believable as possible. Number two: if you know you need a relaxer, don't go and buy no bone-straight ponytail and put that thing on yo' head. That just make a sista talk about you even when she try not to. You know how sometimes you feel all godly, and you say something crazy like "You know I hate to talk about people, but why she didn't relax her head before she put that ponytail on it? Her head looks a mess! I'm sorry, I didn't want to say nothin', but girl, she wrong fa-that."

Number three: if yo hair is black, please don't be walking around with no blonde ponytail. It ain't cute. Not at all. Please try to match up the hair along with yo' ponytail. Please, ladies, we gotta take a little more pride in the way a girl choose her hair buddies like humans. Some of them ain't yo' friend; them things mess up a sista sometimes!

Karen's over there cracking up. "Girl, you know I'm telling the truth. Some of them girls make me just want to fix their hair wherever I see them. I truly have to get myself to turn my head and look at something else. For real, girl, I ain't lying. It's hard on me."

Look, one year, I did a write-up on Professional Women Day for the *Slidell Sentry* newspaper. It was on being aware of your appearance and the message that it delivers to others. I know we, as colored folks, have a bad habit of saying, "I don't care what people think about me!" I'm here to tell you that you better care what people think about you!

See, colored people don't realize, unfortunately, we are prejudged all the time. Our looks: ghetto, uppity, homie, and many more. We do this on a daily basis. Why, I don't know. Whether it makes us feel better to judge others, better than in our moments of sorrows. I want to say when we get ourselves ready to go apply for a job, remember; it matters what you look like, unless it's a black establishment where it's okay to wear these wild three-in-one styles. Sister, it's not accepted on many jobs: the big, hard, high-attention-getter hairstyles. It's not something other cultures want to look at daily. They will prejudge you and the job that you applied for—that you was capable of doing. You won't be given the opportunity to do it because of your appearance.

So drop that craziness: you don't care what people think about you. You better stay conscious about your appearance when you have a plan in life to walk into a job of your dreams. You will always be judged by that look of choice. It tells many stories without one word. I know we are very creative people but you always have to stay aware that we are like guests in this country and people who stand out are not always taken the way we mean for them to be. One hairstyle in a place of business can cause so much discomfort to people of different cultures. We know an afro has been around for years, but it meant power in the black communities. Do you think a brother can get an office job applying with a big afro or corn rows? Some people are uncomfortable being in the presence of our people with these normal cultural looks that we see daily. They find it frightening.

After I wrote that article, I had people walking up to me who I did not know, asking me when I was going to do another write-up. Do you know that next year, after the paper went out, somebody walked up to me and said, "You was the first article I read, and girl, I thought about it all day long." That's what I want as a salon therapist/stylist. I want to make an impact on what people feel and do around me.

Glorious Hair

I pull my big hair up reaching high into the sky.
I pick my tight nappy beautiful hair out as far as I can pick it. Pride is what I feel,
fear is what I inflict.

Glorious Hair

I'm told in my circle of family my hair is my Glory, braided, jheri-curl, or just dreaded down my back. I can't seem to be accepted into this straight-hair world.

Glorious Hair

Listen, my extended family members, Adam and Eve, the original parents to us all, would have loved all their children, nappy-headed, curly-headed and their straight-haired children.

People learn to love the artistic talent of God Almighty for He knew we as people love to be different. So my sista, my brother, don't look at my fro as a gun aimed at you nor my braided hair as a weapon of mass destruction. It's only my Glorious Hair, showing my pride of all the things God blesses me to perform on my crown of Glory.

Glorious Hair!

15

Lord, You Showed up at the Shop Today

Well the sun looks like it's going to do something a little bit this afternoon. So things might just be all right for the folks going to the concert tonight. I'm so glad my girl Sonya is going with her special friend. I'm so happy, Lord, that you moved her today to release some of that pain she has been carrying around with her.

I start talking to God in my mind about Sonya. Lord, you know it's her turn to be happy. Sonya has been through so much. Her life has been so sad. I just want to see her happy. That would be something good for this community to talk about: how Sonya has changed her life, how good she looks, and how wonderful it is that someone came into her life to love her and help her be the wonderful person she truly is. I *love* that girl. She truly is something and I love having her around. People forget what she has been through and sit and talk about her sometimes, but you know we need to stop that. A hard life can make people do things they wouldn't normally do, but because they had no one there to show them how to be a lady, they walk down the wrong road. Now, does that give us the go-ahead to continually make them miserable? No, it don't. People should try and help her by talking to the person or showing some concern for that person, but no, that's too much like right. We have to drag them down more so. God bless her! I think after I finish Karen's hair and nobody shows up, I'm-a close early today and give myself a break. Especially after how my morning got started: falling down in my front yard like somebody crazy. I think that's just what I need. I guess I'll call my daughter, who was supposed to be here right about now getting her hair done, and tell her she better come on here before I leave. Then the two of us can hang out, which means I'll be spending more money then I want to.

I call this child of mind and she talking about she was on her way! Baby, you about to get left without a clean head if you don't come on here.

She asks me just what I knew would get around in my house quick as soon as the kids got up. "Mama, how you fell down this morning? Daddy said you slipped down in the mud this morning and tore up the front yard"

"Oh yeah? Ya'll got jokes today. You better hurry up and get here or yo' messy daddy gonna be doing yo' head. Now, laugh at that! 'Ha ha' that, Miss Thang. I got to go since you trying to be funny."

Yeah, I tore my butt up out there this morning. I don't know what brought that on but you know what? I'm so glad my neighbors just wasn't outside. I can deal with these knuckleheads.

"Well, Karen, you can come on let me rinse your hair out and put you under the dryer so we can get you out of here and you can enjoy the rest of the afternoon."

Karen says, "Girl, yeah, I'ma find something to do with myself, even if it's just the mall. I'm hanging today. Me and Miss Lexus hittin' the streets today."

"Yall gonna do like me and my little missy: find something to do. Since the shop isn't busy, once I do her hair, I guess I'll take her butt to a late lunch. This color came out nice on you. The red is just enough that when the sun hit your head it's going to shine a pretty reddish-brown. Go girl! You gonna be cute today in that mall or wherever ya'll find ya'll selves. All right baby, come sit under this dryer, which I know you hate to do. Take this magazine and relax a minute." I look out the window and see my child pulling up. "Good. Come on here so we can hit the streets."

Nicole walks in and Karen asks, "That's your pretty daughter? She is beautiful." We thank her. Nicole is so shy, she barely opens her mouth when she speaks. She don't mean any harm. My kids are just so quiet. They drive me nuts when I'm talking to them.

"Come on, girl. Sit down at this shampoo bowl. Let me wash this hair. I'm-a just flat iron it and add a little body to it with a medium curling iron. That way you can wrap it tonight."

"I don't want that. I brought me some hair. I want twists with a ponytail."

"Girl, look, don't start. I ain't staying in here all day working on you and that ponytail of yours. I'm telling you now!"

This child thinks all I ever want to do is play in her hair. She can sit there and want this and that taking up my time. Not today.

"All right, I'm do that little ponytail and that's it, okay!"

"Ouch, Mama! You scrubbing my head too hard!"

"Look girl, don't get started. You know you have dandruff and I need to clean your scalp. So, don't start, sista."

"Well, I ain't gonna have a scalp when you get finished."

"Well, I'll scrub yo' eyebrow for you then."

"Yeah, right!"

"Look, get up and get yo' butt in my chair so I can comb through that head of yours. Miss Lexus, I'ma get you in a minute baby. I'ma make sure you are cute as pie. You hear?"

Nicole says, "I want to be cute as pie too."

"Oh girl, you gonna take too long," I say, and Lexus laughs.

Once everybody is finished and my day is now over I grab my bag and run out the door before the next client decides to catch me. As I step out the door, I turn to look inside the shop and it crosses my mind just what all happened today with so few clients. Today was a day the shop was used for God. These are the days when I know God is real. God shows up whereever He is invited and in this salon we are always lifting up His name. Today seems like it was for Sonya herself. It was a day to release, a day to lay her burdens down and be renewed.

"In this little place," I think to myself as I slowly close the door.

Nicole decides to drop her car off at home and to the mall we go. I need a few pictures for the wall. After Hurricane Katrina, we are still decorating the house all over.

16

How Time Fly's

My weekend went so fast, I almost have to be reminded that we had a Sunday and a Monday. It's Tuesday morning again, which means gotta go make the bacon. My little two days passed so fast. I hop into my car, headed to work, when I come across the cutest little white dog.

Oh Lord, you know I can't leave this poor puppy out here to get hit by a car. I could not live with myself. So here I go, out here in the traffic, calling this little pooch who ain't thinking about me. She's looking like, "Honey, I don't know who you calling, but I ain't coming to you!"

"I'm getting tired, Miss Pooch. You better come on here." Okay, let me get my lunch, put some down to see if that will get her. I break a piece of my roast beef sandwich and I guess she smells the roast beef and turns to me like, "Should I or not?" and switched her little self over to enjoy my sandwich. I bent down and scooped her up.

Once I'm home with this little pooch, I get my son to take her and make a couple of signs to see if we can find the owners. God knows I don't need to keep her around. I love dogs, but another one, we don't need. Queen, my little grand-puppy is enough. So, back on the road. I go to my sweet little beauty shop and I think, today I'll do a little spring cleaning if it's not busy. I pull up to the shop and nobody's here. So I run inside, put my things down, and just enjoy the quiet-ness. I love when I come to the salon and nobody's here. It gives me a spiritual moment between me and God.

I decided to leave the shop quiet and do a little cleaning. I love it when it's like this. Sometimes when a client walks into the shop, finding me in here with noth-ing going on and nobody in here, they make the remark, "Oh, it's empty today." Little do they know this salon has been so busy with me and God. I use this time to pray and get myself back in line. I do my humming and singing: at least the words to the song I remember. God and I have the shop packed. If people could see all the spirit that was in this shop, they would never say I'm alone.

Now my peace is over. Here come two cars at one time. Sonya is one of them, with somebody in the car with her. I don't know the other person pulling up, but it's nice to serve new clients anyway.

"Oh look! Here comes my girl I haven't seen in a while, Michelle. I guess I better turn the music on and get myself ready. The quiet day is over." I am surprised to see Sonya back. She was just here Saturday. It must have been a crazy night after the concert.

"Hey ya'll! Come on in. Well, Miss Sonya, what are you doing back so early in the week? Girl, you look like you glowing or something. What's going on with yah, Miss Thang?"

"D, you not going to believe me when I tell you what has happened to me, 'cause I can't believe it. We get to the concert, and girl, our seats are at the front row in front of the stage. Girl, after Maze sang "We Are One," girl, they said, "We would like to thank and welcome a dear friend of our group, Mr. Derrick DeBoise, who is here in town on business along with a beautiful young lady, Miss Sonya Lambert." Derrick stands up and walks towards the stage, he walks up the stairs and onto the stage. I'm like, 'Oh God, what is he about to do?' Derrick takes the microphone and the band starts playing music. Derrick starts singing to me. I thought I was going to pass out. The light shined on me as he sang this beautiful love song to me. Once he was finished singing he asked the crowd did they mind him taking a few minutes to show a very special lady just how much she meant to him.

"Girl, he looked at me he said, 'Sonya, when I saw you for the first time, I knew I had to do whatever it took to meet you. When I saw you and walked up to you to introduce myself to you, you extended your warm, sweet hand to me. My heart felt as if it finally started beating properly, my mind began to make a plan, my body didn't want to move: just be there in your presence. The Sonya I've come to know, the good and the troubled young lady that was, I say: this day, if you would have me, I promise to love you with all my heart from this day until one of us leaves this earth.' He said, 'Sonya, you remind me of a delicate blackberry that's bruised and no one wants to pick it, thinking it's damaged. These are the sweetest berries there is, so ripe and ready to be picked, full of sweetness. Many never experience it because of its appearance, yet it holds the best flavor. I've come to this blackberry patch called New Orleans and I've picked one of the sweetest berries there is. Many people who know you may say many things about your past, the bruised Sonya. The Sonya I know is full of ripeness, sweetness that I want to have forever. Miss Sonya Lambert will you marry me?'

"I couldn't speak for a while until Monica hit my arm and said 'Girl, answer that man!' I started crying and of course, they had those cameras on me, which showed up on the big screen. I shook my head, yes, 'cause I could not speak. Me, Sonya Lambert. This was finally happening. Something good, something a girl only dreams about. I could feel the tears flowing down my face like a waterfall. God was with me. He heard my cry after all. He was giving to me all that I could have dreamed. Me! I just kept thinking: me, out of all these women in this Super-dome. He was allowing this wonderful man to feel this way, when I don't have nothing to give in return.

"Derrick walked down and took me into his arms while the band began another song, which I think we hugged throughout the song until Monica broke the ice and said something crazy, 'Y'all at a concert. Sit down.' We laughed and took our seats. After the concert, we went to the W Hotel where Derrick was staying while he was in town. Derrick opened the door and red roses was every-where: on the floor, on the bed, on the tables, everywhere. I couldn't walk into the room for looking at the beauty. Candles filled the room with sweet spices. The glow from the lit candles was so warm and welcoming. I walked in and noticed a picnic on the middle of the floor. There, he'd had the servers bring in strawberries, chocolate, and whipped cream. We took our shoes off and slipped onto the floor. Derrick dipped a strawberry into the chocolate and brought it to my mouth. It was the sweetest-tasting strawberry I had ever had. He bit off the same berry, than softly kissed my lips, gently touching my face, looking into my eyes like I was the only person in this world.

"My insides was flipping. I didn't know if I could hold down the strawberry that I had. I started to turn my head to take the pressure off me, but he took my face in his hand and told me he didn't care what my life was before him. The per-son God showed him I am is all that mattered. I wanted to say something, 'cause you know, I just don't feel like I have much to offer like he does. He's got a won-derful job, he's a great person. What do I have, but me? It was if he read my mind, because he told me all my attributes. Of course the tears started again. Derrick asked me to stay the night. He had gotten a room adjoined to his. We got up to walk to the room and he said I needed to be able to take a deep hot bath and relax in my new world. When he opened the room door, there, on the bed, lay a single white rose. 'How sweet,' I thought. Derrick asked me, did I know why he gave me a white rose. He said, 'Sonya, if you believe with your heart that Jesus is the Son of God, you shall be saved.' I said 'I do.' He said, 'Then God has wiped away your sin and white stands for pure. You are made whole again, my dear lady.' I walked into the room and Derrick gently kissed me good night.

"When that door closed, girl, I started praising God. I know only God did this. The funny thing was, as I was gettin' my shout on, I heard him saying, 'Thank you, Jesus.' I knew he was truly the one. I walked into the bathroom and looked around at the beauty. Derrick had thought of everything: there was a silk robe lying across a chair, and slippers of the same red color. I stared into the mirror at this blessed girl before stepping into my deep hot tub of water, filled with the sweetest bubbles you could imagine. I just laid there until the water got cold, then I slipped into that beautiful red robe. I didn't put the slippers on because I wanted to feel the deep carpet between my toes. I climbed into this grand bed and when I pulled the covers back, there lay a diamond so big I couldn't believe what I was seeing. I grabbed that ring and ran out that room. He was waiting on me to pull that cover back and find that ring. I couldn't take it no more! I kissed that man like I wanted his soul to come into mine. Girl, I know he was shocked, but I had held my cool long enough. God, I just love this man. He walked me back to my room. It took everything in our body to do the right thing. So I took myself back into the room, but I could not go to sleep. Sleep was the last thing on my mind. I wanted this moment recorded. I wanted to show every moment to someone to help me believe this did happen. D, I look at this ring and I still can't believe these wonderful things are happening!"

"Oh, Sonya! Oh, my God! I am so, so happy for you! Wait, I got to call my husband. I want him to bring champagne. We gonna celebrate right now, then we'll celebrate at the bachelorette party that we will have. Oh, my God, you did it!"

About the Author

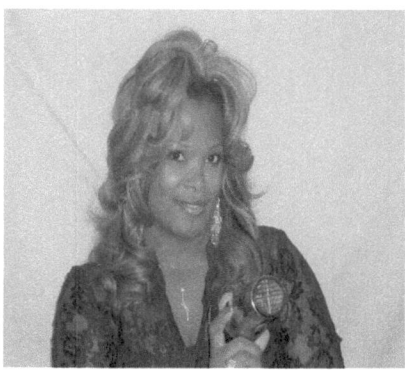

I was born Denise Thompson in the small town of Bogalusa, Louisiana, to a single mother, Lucille Thompson. I was raised in Slidell, Louisiana, by two strong women: my mother and my grandmother, Mattie Thompson-Maiben. This small town was a very close-knit community and I received lots of extra love and nurturing.

I grew up with a strong belief in God, and was taught to pray about everything. I found myself unable to complete high school due to the teenage difficulties of not knowing who I was or where I belonged. Then, while attending John Jay's Beauty College, I found my niche. After sixteen years in my career as a cosmetologist, I've realized there's more in store for me in this field—on a different level. I've always been one to reach out to help someone, and in this field of work God has placed me in a situation where he can use me to deliver his word to people who are hurting and feeling lost.

Writing has always been a way for me to express what I'm feeling, which has made it a good way for me to help someone else. In my marriage to my husband, Eric, and while raising our three kids, writing has given me relief during the heavy and confusing moments.

I'm currently living in Slidell, Louisiana, where I've built many great relationships with my clients. My pastor preached on "walking onto new territory": today I'm taking that walk.

978-0-595-45731-1
0-595-45731-2

www.ingramcontent.com/pod-product-compliance
Lightning Source LLC
Chambersburg PA
CBHW051449280526
45785CB00003B/1492